Palgrave Science Fiction and Fantasy: A New Canon

Series Editors
Sean Guynes
Independent Scholar
Ann Arbor, USA

Keren Omry
Department of English
University of Haifa
Haifa, Israel

Palgrave Science Fiction and Fantasy: A New Canon provides short introductions to key works of science fiction and fantasy (SFF) speaking to why a text, trilogy, or series matters to SFF as a genre as well as to readers, scholars, and fans. These books aim to serve as a go-to resource for thinking on specific texts and series and for prompting further inquiry. Each book will be less than 30,000 words and structured similarly to facilitate classroom use. Focusing specifically on literature, the books will also address film and TV adaptations of the texts as relevant. Beginning with background and context on the text's place in the field, the author and how this text fits in their oeuvre, and the socio-historical reception of the text, the books will provide an understanding of how students, readers, and scholars can think dynamically about a given text. Each book will describe the major approaches to the text and how the critical engagements with the text have shaped SFF. Engaging with classic works as well as recent books that have been taken up by SFF fans and scholars, the goal of the series is not to be the arbiters of canonical importance, but to show how sustained critical analysis of these texts might bring about a new canon. In addition to their suitability for undergraduate courses, the books will appeal to fans of SFF.

Kara Kennedy

Frank Herbert's *Dune*

A Critical Companion

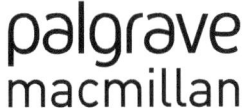

Kara Kennedy
Auckland, New Zealand

ISSN 2662-8562   ISSN 2662-8570 (electronic)
Palgrave Science Fiction and Fantasy: A New Canon
ISBN 978-3-031-13934-5   ISBN 978-3-031-13935-2 (eBook)
https://doi.org/10.1007/978-3-031-13935-2

© The Author(s), under exclusive licence to Springer Nature Switzerland AG 2022
This work is subject to copyright. All rights are solely and exclusively licensed by the Publisher, whether the whole or part of the material is concerned, specifically the rights of translation, reprinting, reuse of illustrations, recitation, broadcasting, reproduction on microfilms or in any other physical way, and transmission or information storage and retrieval, electronic adaptation, computer software, or by similar or dissimilar methodology now known or hereafter developed.
The use of general descriptive names, registered names, trademarks, service marks, etc. in this publication does not imply, even in the absence of a specific statement, that such names are exempt from the relevant protective laws and regulations and therefore free for general use.
The publisher, the authors, and the editors are safe to assume that the advice and information in this book are believed to be true and accurate at the date of publication. Neither the publisher nor the authors or the editors give a warranty, expressed or implied, with respect to the material contained herein or for any errors or omissions that may have been made. The publisher remains neutral with regard to jurisdictional claims in published maps and institutional affiliations.

This Palgrave Macmillan imprint is published by the registered company Springer Nature Switzerland AG.
The registered company address is: Gewerbestrasse 11, 6330 Cham, Switzerland

To all those who have gladly lost themselves in another world

Series Editor's Preface

The infinite worlds of science fiction and fantasy (SFF) dance along the borders between the possible and the impossible, the familiar and the strange, the immediate and the ever-approaching horizon. Speculative fiction in all its forms has been considered a genre, a medium, a mode, a practice, a compilation of themes or a web of assertions. With this in mind, *Palgrave Science Fiction and Fantasy: A New Canon* offers an expansive and dynamic approach to thinking SFF, destabilizing notions of the canon, so long associated with privilege, power, class, and hegemony. We take canon not as a singular and unchallenged authority but as shifting and thoughtful consensus among an always-growing collective of readers, scholars, and writers.

The cultural practice and production of speculation has encompassed novels, stories, plays, games, music, comics, and other media, with a lineage dating back at least to the nineteenth-century precursors through to the most recent publications. Existing scholarship has considered some of these media extensively, often with particular focus on film and TV. It is for this reason that *Palgrave Science Fiction and Fantasy* will forgo the cinematic and televisual, aspiring to direct critical attention at the other nodes of SFF expression.

Each volume in the series introduces, contextualizes, and analyzes a single work of SFF that ranges from the acknowledged "classic" to the should-be-classic, and asks two basic, but provocative questions: *Why does this text matter to SFF? and Why does (or should) this text matter to SFF readers, scholars, and fans?* Thus, the series joins into conversation with both scholars and students of the field to examine the parameters of SFF studies and the changing valences of fundamental categories like genre, medium, and canon. By emphasizing the critical approaches and major questions each text inspires, the series aims to offer "go-to" books for thinking about, writing on, and teaching major works of SFF.

Haifa, Israel   Karen Omry
Ann Arbor, MI   Sean Gynes

Contents

1	**Introduction**	1
	Place in Science Fiction	3
	Cultural Impact	5
	Herbert's Life	6
	Herbert's Other Works	9
	Historical Context	11
	References	15
2	**Power, Politics, and Religion**	19
	Feudalism	20
	Imperialism	21
	Machiavellianism	24
	Religion	27
	Political Systems	31
	References	32
3	**Ecology and the Environment**	35
	The Science of Ecology	36
	The Environment and People	38
	The Ecologist	40
	The Hero	44
	Ecological Science Fiction	45
	References	46

4	Mind and Consciousness	49
	Characterization	50
	Human Potential	52
	Soft Science Fiction	60
	References	61
5	Heroes and Masculinity	63
	Archetypal Hero	64
	Departure from the Archetype	68
	Limitations of the Hero	70
	Criticism of Heroes	72
	Complex Heroes	74
	References	76
6	Women's Influence and Control	77
	Religious Agency	78
	Embodied Agency	81
	Political Agency	84
	The Hero's Debt	87
	Feminist Speculation	87
	References	88
7	A Complex World	89
	References	95
Bibliography		97
Index		109

List of Figures

Fig. 1.1 Paul and Chani in the desert with the Atreides green and black banner and Fremen followers. *Reproduced with permission from illustrator Arthur Whelan*   13

Fig. 2.1 Baron Vladimir Harkonnen fleeing from the poison released by his prisoner, Duke Leto Atreides. *Reproduced with permission from illustrator Arthur Whelan*   25

Fig. 3.1 Fremen planting grasses on dunes. *Reproduced with permission from illustrator Arthur Whelan*   42

Fig. 4.1 Fremen riding the giant sandworm using maker hooks. *Reproduced with permission from illustrator Arthur Whelan*   59

Fig. 5.1 Feyd-Rautha Harkonnen and Paul Atreides face-off in a knife fight. *Reproduced with permission from illustrator Arthur Whelan*   66

Fig. 6.1 A Bene Gesserit woman using the Voice. *Reproduced with permission from illustrator Arthur Whelan*   83

CHAPTER 1

Introduction

Abstract This chapter describes *Dune*'s place in science fiction as a literary work of art with classic themes, a memorable desert landscape, and messages about ecology that remain interesting and relevant. It explains how the book was part of a shift in the genre of science fiction and had a large impact due to its commercial success and its influence on many stories that followed, including *Star Wars*. The chapter also provides an overview of Herbert's influences and interests and draws comparisons between *Dune* and his other works to show that he developed similar themes before and after his masterpiece. It ends with a brief discussion of the historical context, providing a background that is helpful in unpacking the complexities in this multi-layered novel.

Keywords Science fiction • Frank Herbert • Fantasy • Ecology • Environment • Mid-twentieth century fiction

Frank Herbert's science fiction novel *Dune* (1965) has long been acknowledged as a literary work of art [1–3]. It marks the birth of the modern period of science fiction when stories became more sophisticated [4, p. 20]. Its density and complexity demand careful attention [4, p. 316]. It has been called a major work in league with Shakespeare's tragedies, with richness, coherence, and an imaginative vision [5, p. 340].

© The Author(s), under exclusive license to Springer Nature
Switzerland AG 2022
K. Kennedy, *Frank Herbert's* Dune, Palgrave Science Fiction and Fantasy: A New Canon,
https://doi.org/10.1007/978-3-031-13935-2_1

Since selling millions of copies and becoming the best-selling science fiction book of all time, *Dune* has maintained its popularity. It still speaks to us today because of its classic themes, such as love, family, loyalty, betrayal, leadership, power, ambition, and culture clashes. It explores concerns about the future, humans' place in the environment, and the fate of civilization. It also makes allusions to ancient mythology, which links it with the epic tradition. For example, House Atreides headed by Duke Leto alludes to the cursed House of Atreus and Leto, the mother of the twins Artemis and Apollo, from Greek mythology [6, 7]. In addition, there are parallels with historical issues that continue to impact us, including tensions between East and West, conflicts over oil, drug usage, human rights, and religion. The book builds a fantastical world that seems believable because it is based on familiar events and landscapes. *Dune* has also avoided becoming dated in part through its focus on humans rather than technology. It gives us characters that are based on classic archetypes but become three-dimensional when we see how they think and what they feel. It offers layers of meaning that reward multiple readings—we can still make surprising discoveries and experience the world in new ways when we return to it. These add the kind of complexity that elevates the book's literary importance. *Dune* has withstood the test of time for many reasons. In this study, we will explore some of the major themes, perspectives, and context that have helped it achieve the status of a masterpiece.

Dune is probably best known for its setting—the desert world of Arrakis, also known as Dune—and for its environmental themes. This harsh, arid landscape filled with giant sandworms captures the imagination. Underpinning the story is the idea that everything is interconnected, which is the basic principle of ecology—the study of interactions between creatures and their environment. The book's publication was timely. The pioneer of the modern environmental movement, biologist Rachel Carson, had recently published *Silent Spring* (1962), and the American public were opening their eyes to the destruction that humans were causing to the planet. It was a prime moment for an epic tale told of a world where the locals who live in harmony with the environment are threatened by greedy off-worlders who care only to mine the planet for a precious resource. In *Dune*, there is a character explicitly named as an ecologist, who leads a secret terraforming project with the locals' assistance to convert the desert into a water-filled paradise. Yet even this scientist neglects to foresee the unintended consequences of such a radical change to the ecosystem. With these elements, both obvious and subtle, *Dune* became a pioneer in ecological science fiction and is credited for helping spur the modern environmental movement.

The U.S. counterculture claimed *Dune* as its own when a book review was published in the *Whole Earth Catalog* in 1968. Now known as the magnum opus of the counterculture, the catalog introduced ideas like organic farming, alternative energy sources, and computers to a mainstream audience [8]. It called *Dune* "rich re-readable fantasy with clear portrayal of the fierce environment it takes to cohere a community. [...] The metaphor is ecology. The theme revolution" [9, p. 41]. Here was a book that could guide people's thinking and warn them of the consequences of humanity's interference with Mother Earth. Herbert commented that he chose the title deliberately to echo the sound of 'doom' [10, p. 249]. *Dune* was hitting the right notes about the environment at the right moment.

It was also discovered by university staff and students, who helped launch it to success. Like J.R.R. Tolkien's *The Lord of the Rings* (1954–1955) and Robert Heinlein's *Stranger in a Strange Land* (1961), *Dune* became a campus book, consumed by hundreds of thousands of students as a countercultural statement [5, p. 337]. Its ecological message and inclusion of a hallucinogenic drug certainly helped fuel its popularity. Some staff adopted it as textbook material for their courses, and by 1974 it was considered one of the most popular books to introduce students to the genre of science fiction [1, 11]. It was also recommended for use in high school English courses [11, pp. 74–75]. *Cliffs Notes on Herbert's Dune and Other Works* was published in 1975, giving further evidence that the book was used enough in education to warrant a study guide. Science fiction was going mainstream, and *Dune* benefited from the trend of this genre moving beyond a dedicated niche of fans [5, p. 337].

PLACE IN SCIENCE FICTION

Dune was published during a time of transition for the relatively young genre of science fiction. The 1950s saw science fiction expanding to reach a broader audience interested in learning about discoveries and technologies such as space exploration and atomic energy [12, p. 80]. Sometimes described as Golden Age science fiction, many stories during the period 1940–1960 featured ideas grounded in recognizable science, linear storylines, and problem-solving heroes [5, p. 287]. Influential writers included Isaac Asimov and Robert Heinlein, who wrote stories that engaged with big ideas and speculated about the potential of technology to create a brighter future, though there were cautionary science fiction tales as well.

Another influential figure was John W. Campbell, editor of the science fiction magazine *Astounding*, later renamed *Analog*. He saw the potential in Herbert's lengthy story and published it in serialized form as "Dune World" (three parts) and "The Prophet of Dune" (five parts) in issues from December 1963 to May 1965. Campbell had strong opinions about what made a good science fiction story, and there is a connection between his personal tastes and the characteristics of Golden Age stories [5, p. 287]. He shaped how authors revised their work for publication, thus making a mark on the path the genre would take. We can see from his correspondence with Herbert that he had a clear idea about how to handle supermen in science fiction, and he believed Herbert was setting up Paul to be too powerful and hard to defeat [10, p. 112]. Herbert disagreed that the story needed a major rewrite, though, and instead made minor changes on other aspects not involving Paul's powers [13, p. 174]. Years later, Campbell would turn down Herbert's submission of a sequel story, *Dune Messiah*, because the editor did not have an interest in showing the hero, Paul, turning into an anti-hero [10, p. 109]. Nonetheless, Campbell validated Herbert's talent, even as Herbert had difficulty finding a book publisher who would take a chance on his long story. Eventually he secured an agreement with Chilton, known for its auto repair manuals, for a hardback edition and then Ace Books, a science fiction publisher, for a paperback. But it still took several years for *Dune* to become a bestseller.

Dune became notable for its world-building and has been held up as a masterpiece alongside Tolkien's fantasy series *The Lord of the Rings* [14, p. 123]. Both develop a variety of new terms, cultures, and factions, as well as the sense that the world expands beyond the borders of the time and space presented in the main storyline. *Dune* proved that science fiction could, like fantasy, take the time to carefully construct a believable world that readers would want to immerse themselves in. A story could be lengthy and include historical context, maps, and appendices that provided additional information without clogging up the storyline. It could leave things unexplained and let the reader fill in the gaps using their imagination [15]. Soon after its publication as a novel, *Dune* won both of the top science fiction awards: it won the Nebula Award for best novel in 1965, given by the Science Fiction and Fantasy Writers of America, and shared the Hugo Award for best novel in 1966, given by the World Science Fiction Society.

Dune was something unique in science fiction. In some ways it resembled stories of the Golden Age; it had elements of more traditional or 'hard' science fiction, such as space travel and explanations of how the science would work on another planet. But it also featured significant interest in humans and human consciousness, which were characteristics of 'soft' science fiction. This was part of the turn that writers such as J.G. Ballard were making toward the exploration of 'inner space,' or human potentiality, and away from a focus on outer space and technological gadgetry. Stories with these types of characteristics were part of the New Wave, the period of the 1960s and 1970s that had some science fiction writers engaging in more experimentation with style and content and explicit language or sexual references [16, p. 103]. With its mixture of styles and themes, *Dune* did not fit neatly into Golden Age or New Wave categories. It explored the role of a messiah in human culture, as did other important 1960s texts such as Heinlein's *Stranger in a Strange Land*, but its hero lacked control over his future path. Some consider *Dune* to be a direct response to Asimov's 1950s *Foundation* series: a critique of its faith in science and the idea that intelligent scientists could predict the future and guide things toward a better state of affairs [5, 17]. Yet what really made *Dune* stand out from the science fiction that had gone before was its attention to detail and its sheer scale [1, 18]. Therefore, *Dune* can best be described as a bridge-builder between different types of science fiction that heralded the maturation of the genre.

Cultural Impact

Part of *Dune*'s legacy is the impact it had as an inspiration for many stories that followed it. These include science fiction—such as Kim Stanley Robinson's *Mars* trilogy (1992–1996) and Joan Slonczewski's *A Door into Ocean* (1986); fantasy—such as Robert Jordan's *The Wheel of Time* series (1990–2013); and anime—such as Carl Macek's *Robotech* television series (1985). The massively influential Star Wars franchise owes *Dune* a significant debt. There are undeniable similarities between *Dune* and *Star Wars: A New Hope* (1977) by director George Lucas, including the desert planet and its inhabitants, character names and characteristics, and philosophies about balance and nature. Herbert and other writers who saw their work in Lucas' film even jokingly created a loose organization called the We're Too Big to Sue George Lucas Society [13, p. 288]. A big concern was the challenge of trying to adapt *Dune* when key concepts had already been used in *Star Wars*. Any screen adaptation might appear to be a mere copy.

Eventually *Dune* would be adapted into film—first by director David Lynch in 1984, and again by director Denis Villeneuve in 2021. The first three novels were also adapted into two television miniseries—*Frank Herbert's Dune* and *Frank Herbert's Children of Dune*—directed by John Harrison and Greg Yaitanes, respectively, in 2000 and 2003. Although these adaptations did not spawn the billion-dollar franchise of Star Wars, they reinvigorated interest in Herbert's story and introduced it to new generations. After Lynch's film, *Dune* reached number one on *The New York Times* bestseller list, and after Villeneuve's adaptation, it once again became a bestseller [13, p. 474]. Even the 1970s film adaptation that was never made, involving director Alejandro Jodorowsky, prompted a creative outpouring that spilled over into other projects, including Ridley Scott's award-winning *Alien* (1979) film [19]. There have also been games, comics, and other books set in the *Dune* universe that draw on the characters and themes from the original book.

Through its threads of influence, *Dune* has played a pivotal role in shaping science fiction during its massive growth in the latter half of the twentieth century and beyond. Its epic nature, depth, and breadth encouraged other writers to pursue more complexity than they might have otherwise [4, pp. 399–400]. In addition, its commercial success paved the way for larger advances, more printings, and higher sales for other science fiction novels, leading to more bestsellers for the genre [20, p. 353]. The book brought awareness of ecology to the center of the genre and shaped the ecological science fiction stories that followed [12, p. 87]. It also elevated world-building and characterization to worthy pursuits in a genre that was often looked down on as not worthy of serious consideration. Decades ago, *Dune* signaled a major shift in science fiction, and it still has a lot left to offer us as a work of literature.

Herbert's Life

Herbert's wide range of interests played an important role in shaping the content and complexity of what would become *Dune*. Born in Tacoma, Washington, on October 8, 1920, Herbert grew up in a rural area, which helped give him the do-it-yourself mentality and respect for the natural environment that is threaded throughout *Dune*. He spent his formative years outdoors on the Olympic and Kitsap peninsulas of northwest

Washington surrounded by forests and water [1, 13, 21]. Although his father was agnostic, his mother was from a Catholic family and her ten sisters insisted Herbert receive Catholic training, which was delivered by Jesuits. We can see reflections of his aunts in the influential women of the Bene Gesserit, who maintain political influence and power in an otherwise male-dominated society. Herbert even described the characters as female Jesuits and gave them a similar-sounding name [13, 21, 22].

As a journalist, Herbert gained skills in research and writing that would come in handy during the years of study he spent in preparation to write his masterpiece. He entered journalism as a teenager at the *Glendale Star* and went on to work for other West Coast newspapers, including the *Oregon Journal*, *Seattle Post-Intelligencer*, and *San Francisco Examiner*. He spent some time in higher education, taking courses on mathematics, psychology, and English at the University of Washington, where he met his second spouse, Beverly Stuart, in a creative writing class [13, p. 56]. He was especially interested in psychology and dabbled some in psychoanalysis. His friendship with psychologists Ralph and Irene Slattery exposed him to Freudian and Jungian theories, as well as Zen Buddhism and the emerging science of nonverbal communication, that would make their way into *Dune* [21, pp. 18–19]. Jungian conceptions of archetypes, the collective unconscious, and masculine and feminine energies can be seen in multiple characters, especially Jessica and Paul.

Herbert's political views are hard to locate on the conventional political spectrum, but what comes across in his writing is his skepticism of governments and bureaucracies. He was not against them completely but was critical of their inefficiencies and tendency to self-perpetuate in a kind of feudal system based on loyalty. Working behind the scenes in politics also helped fuel Herbert's criticisms regarding the inner mechanisms of government, including the tactics politicians use to influence others. In the 1950s he worked on the staff of several Republican candidates for office in Oregon and Washington, including Senator Guy Cordon. As part of his role as a researcher and political speechwriter for Cordon, Herbert traveled to the U.S. Senate's Army-McCarthy hearings in 1954 and saw firsthand the inquiry into Americans suspected of communist sympathies. Herbert himself was a distant cousin of Senator Joseph McCarthy, the leader of the campaign, and saw where the obsession with security and control could lead [21, p. 35]. As a writer, he was well aware of the power of language to shape people's thinking, and in *Dune* he includes several politically savvy characters who leverage language to play politics and influence those around them. His interest in language was also influenced by his work in general semantics, a linguistics philosophy concerned with the need for more scientific and careful use of language and communication. He studied it in San Francisco around the same time as writing *Dune*, and worked as a ghostwriter for the popular general semantics advocate S.I. Hayakawa [21, pp. 59–60]. General semantics finds its way into the Bene Gesserit's operations and philosophy and the broader theme of the power of language to manipulate others.

Although Herbert later gained fame for his environmentalist work, this came after the success of *Dune*. The book shows us the seeds of his interest in ecology and humans' impact on nature. In his telling, the inspiration for *Dune* originated when he was tasked with writing a story about the U.S. Department of Agriculture's work to control the sand dunes in Oregon through a natural method of planting grass rather than building a wall [21, p. 39]. This then provided an idea for a story merging ecology with a major theme he had been pondering: people's tendency to follow leaders or messiahs, who had historically often emerged from a desert environment.

Herbert's emerging skepticism of Westerners' impact on the environment was likely influenced by his friendships with two men who had lived on the Native American reservation of the Quileute Nation in Washington: Henry Martin and Howard Hansen [23]. A member of the Hoh, a small group of Quileute people, Martin was a fisher who found himself displaced due to outside pressures and sometime in his forties met a young Herbert who was out fishing [23, p. 195]. They became friends and Martin taught Herbert valuable skills related to hunting, fishing, and living off the land [13, p. 31]. We can see this influence in several of Herbert's stories that feature "whites, usually boys, befriending Native men," such as happens with Paul and Stilgar in *Dune* [23, p. 197]. Hansen had also lived on the Quileute reservation, although he was not an officially enrolled member. He was a teenager when he met Herbert just after World War II, and they became best friends. As an emerging writer and environmentalist, Hansen warned of the planet being turned into a wasteland by white men [23]. Both Martin and Hansen provided Herbert with an alternate view of imperialism and modernization and ideas for what would become his ecological warning to the world.

Also integral to Herbert's work was his spouse, Beverly, whom he married after his first brief marriage to Flora Parkinson, with whom he had a daughter, Penny. A fellow writer, Beverly worked as an advertising copywriter and supported Herbert's interest in writing science fiction. She took on the role of breadwinner when he took breaks from journalism to pursue his writing career, and he would take care of their sons, Brian and Bruce, and the house [21, p. 17]. As with many writing couples, we cannot know the full extent to which they worked together and assisted each other in the writing process. But Brian has acknowledged her pivotal role in editing Herbert's manuscripts, making suggestions, and helping with plot and characterization, especially the motivation of female characters [13, p. 138, 170]. Beverly was Herbert's partner for almost four decades, and we can see from Herbert's words—"She's the best thing that ever happened to me"—and the dedications in the later *Dune* novels that she was deeply loved and valued by him, and her passing from cancer in 1984 affected him greatly [21, p. 17]. Combined with the influence from his mother and ten maternal aunts, women's impact was strong in Herbert's life and arguably one reason for the presence of feminist themes in *Dune* before the second-wave feminist movement had gained momentum [24, p. 3].

Herbert's Other Works

Dune is Herbert's masterpiece, but it is not the only science fiction story he wrote and published. In his earlier works, we can see him working out some of the themes that would make their way into *Dune* in more fully fleshed form.

We can find several similarities between Herbert's second novel, *Dune*, and his first novel, *The Dragon in the Sea* (1956), also known as *21st Century Sub* or *Under Pressure*. In this submarine thriller, Herbert explores the psychological workings of a crew of four as they try to uncover an enemy sleeper agent in their midst and avoid being sabotaged and killed like the previous twenty expeditions. The story highlights the psychological adaptations that humans make to their living conditions and larger social conditions [25, p. 72]. Herbert uses italicized text to show the internal mental workings of several characters, just as he does in *Dune*. He switches between the third-person narrator, characters' thoughts, and dialogue to give different perspectives on events and how humans process them. He also mentions concepts that appear in *Dune*, including Jungian psychology and ecology. On a broader level, the Cold War concern between East and West appears with the crew being Americans and the enemy being the Eastern Powers, which includes Russia. There is a resource scarcity regarding oil, and each nation is prepared to invest significant resources to obtain and secure it. Since its setting is largely limited to the submarine, though, *The Dragon in the Sea* does not offer the same wide cast of characters, including female ones, or expansive world development that features in *Dune*.

Herbert's strong interest in psychology underpins many of his works. This is arguably one reason stories such as *Dune* have withstood the test of time. We continue to be interested in ourselves and how we think, even as the gadgets and technology change around us. Themes surrounding the mind and awareness, Jungian concepts of memory and the unconscious, and psi powers, including prescience, appear in many of Herbert's stories, including *Dune*. One story, "The Priests of Psi" (1960), has parallels with *Dune* in that it features a man being tested by religious leaders interested in his psychic powers, just as Paul Atreides is tested by the Bene Gesserit. Lewis Orne encounters psi awareness, prescient warnings, and a psi machine not unlike the Bene Gesserit's black box of pain. He must practice focus and calming regimes as Paul does, and he learns about the science of religion and how the priests find and educate prophets in the hope of containing or redirecting religion's explosive energy. This is similar to what the Bene Gesserit attempt, though it is less explicitly stated in *Dune*. Herbert expanded upon Orne's story in *The Godmakers* (1972), which has the hero's journey, an organization of women with skills in politics and reproductive control, and the messianic impulse that all appear in *Dune* [25, p. 62, 72]. In these as well as other works, Herbert examines the nature of gods and how they are created, and the consequences for the universe, such as religious-inspired violence, when a human takes on such a powerful role [25, p. 62].

Another common feature in Herbert's stories is concealment [3, p. 81]. Characters may hide information or have hidden powers, traitors or saboteurs may be unknown, and communities may hold secrets. There are also often ideas relating to ecology and the adaptation to new environments in Herbert's works. A frequent theme revolves around humans' reactions to different kinds of change in their world [25, p. 17]. Herbert looks at humans' place in the ecosystem, showing that they are not set apart and need to be cautious about trying to change systems. He also examines the process of getting along with others who are different, whether they be people, artificial intelligence, or insects [25, p. 27]. A major theme that appears throughout his works is the use of power, particularly how governments use it, and ways to subvert that power or limit its effects [25, p. 22]. Reproduction and genetic manipulation play a role in this theme as well.

Despite similarities in themes, however, none of Herbert's other works meets the scope or reaches the level of complexity of *Dune*. This is his literary masterpiece that brings together many threads and interweaves them into a multi-layered and interesting blend of storytelling, lessons, and warnings. Herbert went on to write five sequels to *Dune*—*Dune Messiah* (1969), *Children of Dune* (1976), *God Emperor of Dune* (1981), *Heretics of Dune* (1984), and *Chapterhouse: Dune* (1985)—making a six-book saga that spans around 3500 years in that universe. These gave him the space to explore the world he set up in the first book and move the storyline in new directions. Themes developed further in the sequels include the nature of humanity, evolution and genetics, prescience in relation to the Atreides line, the influence of the Bene Gesserit, tyranny and subservience, religious fervor, and the environment. Throughout the series, Herbert is increasingly explicit in his critique of heroes and shows Paul forced to come to terms with the negative consequences of his actions in *Dune*. There are new enemies to replace Baron Harkonnen and Emperor Shaddam IV, new settings, and new challenges, but much of the story still revolves around the planet Dune and who holds the reins of power.

HISTORICAL CONTEXT

As with many science fiction authors, Herbert responded to the issues of his time by adapting and projecting them into a new, fantastical environment to both entertain readers and prompt them to consider their world in a new light. Part of what keeps *Dune* relevant is that many of the historical issues present during the 1950s and 1960s remain issues today. Although we can certainly enjoy the book without knowing much about these issues, being more aware of the social and historical context in which it was written can help deepen our understanding and appreciation of the many facets of this science fiction classic.

The post-World War II period saw the U.S. benefit from its position of global leadership and take a greater interest in international relations and affairs. High on its victory over the Axis nations, the country rebounded from the Great Depression and entered a period of economic prosperity and growth. But the threat of fascism was soon replaced with the perceived threat of communism, which had spread after the October Revolution in Russia in 1917 and the establishment of the Soviet Union five years later. Tensions between the Soviet Union and the U.S. escalated in what would become known as the Cold War, a nuclear stand-off that dominated global politics for nearly fifty years and was fought in proxy wars across the globe, including in Korea and Vietnam. These tensions appeared in various forms of popular culture. Villains were often coded as Russian, as Baron Harkonnen in *Dune* is through his first name, Vladimir, and nuclear weapons were used in fictional military maneuvers, as when Paul deploys the family atomics against the Shield Wall.

During this time, the Middle East grew in importance as oil became an increasingly valuable substance for industrialized nations. This petroleum-rich region became a strategic battleground between the Democratic West and Communist East. The Eisenhower Doctrine of 1957 pledged the U.S. to send armed forces there to protect nations against communist aggression. Foreign companies had controlled a majority of petroleum production and distribution in the region, but locals began seeking a larger percentage of the profits. In 1960, the Organization of the Petroleum Exporting Countries (OPEC)—initially comprising Saudi Arabia, Iraq, Iran, Kuwait, and Venezuela—was founded to gain more control over oil prices. There would be many parallels with this situation in Herbert's depiction of the deserts of Arrakis and conflict over the valuable resource of spice.

Otherwise, the Middle East was still often perceived as an exotic place in a far-away desert populated by tent-dwelling Arabs, as depicted in the award-winning film *Lawrence of Arabia* (1962). This immensely popular film showed British officer T.E. Lawrence helping lead the Arabs against the Ottoman Turks, who were allied with Germany and the other Central Powers during World War I. The story was based on Lawrence's war memoir, *Seven Pillars of Wisdom* (1926), which Herbert read before writing *Dune* [13, p. 141]. In general, popular culture portrayed Arabs as stereotypically violent and uncivilized outsiders who were to be feared or defeated [26]. Basing his Fremen characters off of Bedouin Arabs as well as other cultures, Herbert offered a more nuanced and complex portrayal of desert dwellers who faced intrusion from outsiders in their lands (see Fig. 1.1).

Another charismatic leader who was popular at this time was John F. Kennedy, who rose through the political ranks as a New England congressperson to be elected president of the U.S. in the November 1960 election. Many Americans fell in love with President Kennedy and the romantic glamor and Camelot-type aura he brought to the White House,

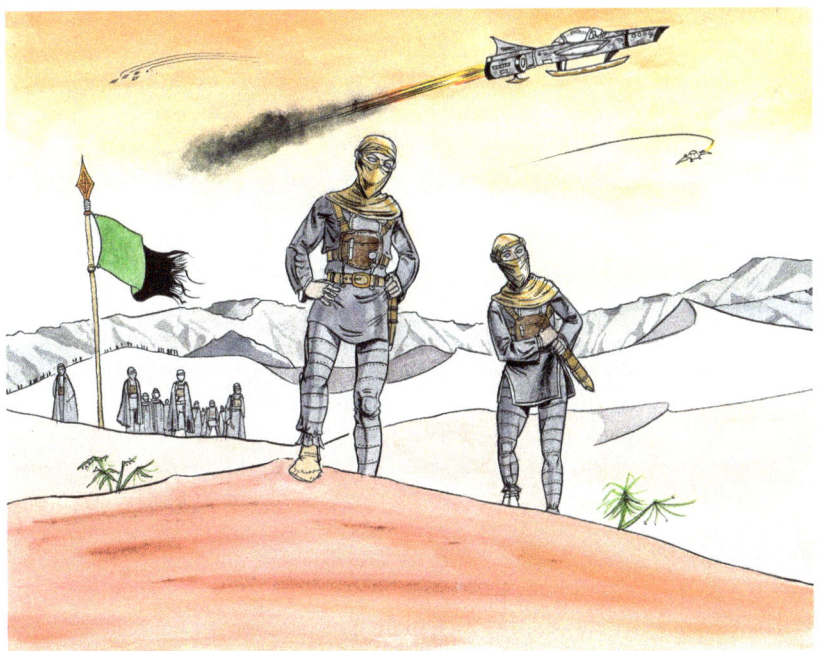

Fig. 1.1 Paul and Chani in the desert with the Atreides green and black banner and Fremen followers. *Reproduced with permission from illustrator Arthur Whelan*

with his stylish spouse, Jacqueline, and charming young children in tow. As the youngest elected president and first Roman Catholic, he represented youthful optimism and hope for change, and his programs were associated with the idea of a New Frontier. This made it all the more devastating for the country when he was assassinated just three years later. Herbert was critical of such charismatic figures, and he specifically named Kennedy as an example of someone who took on a larger-than-life, mythic status that convinced people to give up their decision-making capacity [10, p. 98]. Echoes of the Kennedy Presidency can be seen in the characterization of House Atreides and Herbert's attempt to warn readers against falling for these heroic figures [27, p. 124].

The postwar period was also a time of massive cultural and social upheaval. The 1950s saw the emergence of the civil rights movement in which many Black Americans and their allies fought against discrimination, persecution, and the ever-present threat of being lynched through a range of tactics, including boycotts, sit-ins, and demonstrations. Meanwhile, influenced by key texts such as French philosopher Simone de Beauvoir's *The Second Sex* (translated in 1953) and American journalist Betty Friedan's *The Feminine Mystique* (1963), many women were gearing up for a large-scale push for equal rights that in the late 1960s would become known as the women's liberation movement, or second-wave feminism. The contraceptive pill was approved by the Food and Drug Administration in 1960, signaling a change in sexual behaviors and paving the way for the sexual revolution. Even the long-standing Catholic Church was undergoing significant changes. The Second Vatican Council (Vatican II) brought together thousands of bishops and other members of the Church between 1962 and 1965 to make decisions about necessary updates to Catholicism.

These conditions contributed to an atmosphere of change and disruption that likely had an influence on Herbert as he was researching for and writing *Dune*. The book highlights clashes between classes and cultures more so than racial tensions, but it taps into the longing of marginalized groups for freedom from oppression and brutality. It draws on Catholic traditions and beliefs for the all-female Bene Gesserit order, and shows these women having significant control and influence. Yet although some postwar issues are noticeably reflected in *Dune*, in other respects the book is predictive science fiction. Issues such as the popular use of hallucinogenic drugs, insatiable demand for a valuable resource found in the desert sands, environmental threats, conflict and religious tensions in the Middle East, and concerns over advanced technologies had yet to fully emerge. Herbert also incorporated elements that were still on the edge of becoming widely known or researched in the U.S., including biofeedback, nonverbal communication, altered states of consciousness, and Eastern disciplines such as Zen Buddhism and Yoga [21, pp. 60–61].

When we encounter *Dune* today, informed by our own historical context, we bring a different perspective to these issues. But we can still recognize their continued relevance. The Cold War may be over, but tensions between Western and Eastern nations continue to rise or fall depending on changes in leadership, foreign policies, and economic conditions. Conflict in the Middle East has been a mainstay of the twentieth and twenty-first centuries, and terrorism has become an everyday word and ever-present threat. The U.S. and other Western countries have spent significant resources engaging in wars or providing assistance to other governments in the region. Concerns over climate change have so far not dampened the demand for oil. The struggle for equal rights and equity for women, people of color, and other marginalized groups continues, with both gains and setbacks. Drugs and their effect on the human mind remain a topic of interest [28]. Hallucinogens such as LSD and psilocybin are again being studied for therapeutic treatment and used in certain circles, and marijuana has been legalized in many places in the U.S. for medical or recreational purposes. The Catholic Church remains influential as the largest religious institution in the U.S., though it has been rocked by priest abuse scandals and coverups that have impacted its reputation. Polls suggest many Catholics would like to see the church relax restrictions on policies such as the ban on birth control, priests not being allowed to marry, and women not being ordained as priests [29]. Technology may have advanced since *Dune*'s publication, but humans are still wrestling with age-old concerns about the future and their fate in the world.

The following chapters unpack some of the many layers of complexity in *Dune* by looking at five different ways of understanding this science fiction classic. Chapter 2 covers power, politics, and the treatment of religion. This includes an exploration of feudalism, imperialism, Machiavellianism, and religion. Chapter 3 covers ecology and the environment, and humans' attempt to control nature rather than conserve it. Chapter 4 explores the themes of the human mind and consciousness. It examines the development of complex and three-dimensional characters who have psychological depth. Chapter 5 looks at the hero archetype in relation to Paul and stereotypical characteristics of masculinity. This covers his strengths and limitations and his role in the book's critique of heroes and messianic figures. Chapter 6 examines the complexity of the representation of women and how they are shown having control and influence. It focuses on religious, embodied, and political avenues of control for women. Chapter 7 concludes by reviewing other ways of interpreting *Dune* and giving food for thought on new avenues for study.

REFERENCES

1. Touponce, William. *Frank Herbert.* Twayne Publishers, 1988.
2. Ower, John. "Idea and Imagery in Herbert's *Dune.*" *Extrapolation*, vol. 15, no. 2, 1974, pp. 129-139.
3. Manlove, C.N. "Frank Herbert, *Dune* (1965)." *Science Fiction: Ten Explorations.* Macmillan Press, 1986, pp. 79-99.

4. Aldiss, Brian, and David Wingrove. *Trillion Year Spree: The History of Science Fiction.* Atheneum, 1986.
5. Roberts, Adam. *The History of Science Fiction.* 2nd ed., Palgrave Macmillan, 2016.
6. Rogers, Brett M. "'Now Harkonnen Shall Kill Harkonnen': Aeschylus, Dynastic Violence, and Twofold Tragedies in Frank Herbert's *Dune.*" *Brill's Companion to the Reception of Aeschylus*, edited by Rebecca Futo Kennedy, Brill, 2018, pp. 553-581.
7. Sloan, Russell. *Evolution, The Messianic Hero, and Ecology in Frank Herbert's Dune Sequence.* 2010. University of Ulster, PhD dissertation.
8. Cadwalladr, Carole. "Stewart Brand's Whole Earth Catalog, the Book that Changed the World." *The Observer*, 5 May 2013. https://www.theguardian.com/books/2013/may/05/stewart-brand-whole-earth-catalog
9. Brand, Stewart. *Whole Earth Catalog.* Fall 1968.
10. Herbert, Frank. *Maker of Dune*, edited by Tim O'Reilly, Berkley Books, 1987.
11. Calkins, Elizabeth, and Barry McGhan. *A Handbook of Science Fiction for Teachers.* Pflaum/Standard, 1972.
12. Latham, Rob. "Biotic Invasions: Ecological Imperialism in New Wave Science Fiction." *Green Planets: Ecology and Science Fiction*, edited by Gerry Canavan and Kim Stanley Robinson, Wesleyan University Press, 2014, pp. 77-95.
13. Herbert, Brian. *Dreamer of Dune: The Biography of Frank Herbert.* Tom Doherty Associates, 2003.
14. Pierce, John J. *Foundations of Science Fiction: A Study in Imagination and Evolution.* Greenwood Press, 1987.
15. Wolf, Mark J.P. *Building Imaginary Worlds: The Theory and History of Subcreation.* Routledge, 2012.
16. Merrick, Helen. "Fiction, 1964–1979." *The Routledge Companion to Science Fiction*, edited by Mark Bould, Andrew Butler, Adam Roberts, and Sherryl Vint, Routledge, 2009, pp. 102–111.
17. Grigsby, John L. "Asimov's 'Foundation' Trilogy and Herbert's 'Dune' Trilogy: A Vision Reversed." *Science Fiction Studies*, vol. 8, no. 2, 1981, pp. 149–155.
18. Aldiss, Brian. *Billion Year Spree: The True History of Science Fiction.* Doubleday, 1973.
19. *Jodorowsky's Dune.* Directed by Frank Pavich, Sony Pictures, 2013.
20. McNelly, Willis E. "In Memoriam: Frank Herbert, 1920–1986." *Extrapolation*, vol. 27, no. 4, 1986, pp. 352–355.
21. O'Reilly, Timothy. *Frank Herbert.* Frederick Ungar, 1981.
22. Kennedy, Kara. "Epic World-Building: Names and Cultures in *Dune.*" *Names*, vol. 64, no. 2, 2016, pp. 99–108.
23. Immerwahr, Daniel. "The Quileute *Dune*: Frank Herbert, Indigeneity, and Empire." *Journal of American Studies*, vol. 56, no. 2, 2022, pp. 191–216.

24. Kennedy, Kara. *Women's Agency in the* Dune *Universe: Tracing Women's Liberation through Science Fiction*. Palgrave Macmillan, 2021.
25. Allen, David L. *Cliffs Notes on Herbert's Dune and Other Works*. Cliffs Notes, 1975.
26. Shaheen, Jack G. *Reel Bad Arabs: How Hollywood Vilifies a People*. Olive Branch Press, 2001.
27. Liddell, Elisabeth, and Michael Liddell. "*Dune*: A Tale of Two Texts." *Cinema and Fiction: New Modes of Adapting, 1950–1990*, edited by John Orr and Colin Nicholson, Edinburgh University Press, 1992, pp. 122–139.
28. Pollan, Michael. *How to Change Your Mind: The New Science of Psychedelics*. Allen Lane, 2018.
29. Pew Research Center. "Expectations of the Church." 2 Sept. 2015, https://www.pewforum.org/2015/09/02/chapter-4-expectations-of-the-church/#catholic-desires-for-change

CHAPTER 2

Power, Politics, and Religion

Abstract This chapter discusses issues of power, politics, and religion in *Dune*, with a focus on the interplay between feudalism, imperialism, and Machiavellianism. It shows how these features are important in the development of a universe that focuses on humans rather than technology, which allows Herbert to highlight the corruption in the strategies of groups seeking control. The chapter also examines the Catholic, Islamic, and Arabic influences on the depiction of religion and the characterization of the Bene Gesserit and Fremen in the book. It discusses these in relation to Herbert's criticism of the potential for religion to be used as a political tool.

Keywords Science fiction • Frank Herbert • Politics • Religion • Catholicism • Islam

Dune invites us to a future that is much like the past. A classical feudal system with dukes and barons in service to an emperor, who must keep the economy running to satisfy the guild and trade organizations while also appeasing the church. An age based on medieval Europe where advanced technology is banned, treachery is accomplished through poison or deceitful household staff, and combat is largely limited to hand-to-hand fights. An exotic land with rich resources and a tribal people who spark curiosity and fear in outsiders. What draws us into this future is the world that Herbert builds around these familiar features. We enter it just as the political tides are shifting, so we want to see how the tensions resolve. In this chapter, we look at the features of power, politics, and religion. We examine the interplay between feudalism, imperialism, and Machiavellianism. And we explore how *Dune* combines real-world political systems and religions in a science fictional context in order to help us reflect on their operations and at-times corruptive influences.

Feudalism

The use of a feudal framework in *Dune* makes the lines of power clear and recognizable [1]. Feudalism also highlights the interconnections between the various factions and how they feed back to each other, which ties into the larger ecological theme. We become aware early on in *Dune* about the major factions and balance of power in the Imperium. This immediately focuses our attention on politics and establishes our understanding of the political ecosystem that is about to become severely disrupted. We learn of the "three-point civilization: the Imperial Household balanced against the Federated Great Houses of the Landsraad, and between them, the Guild" and "feudal trade culture which turns its back on most science" [2, p. 23]. The Imperial Household is comprised of the Padishah Emperor Shaddam IV of House Corrino and his five daughters. His title includes the Persian *padishah*, meaning 'master king,' and links him with the historic Persian rulers and Ottoman sultans [3]. The Landsraad consists of noble houses headed by leaders such as Duke Leto of House Atreides and Baron Vladimir of House Harkonnen. Its Scandinavian name, meaning Parliament or Land Council, reminds us that land is essential to being part of the nobility and having access to decision-making power [4, p. 121]. The Spacing Guild maintains a monopoly on interstellar space travel through its navigators' special ability to pilot ships with the aid of spice. The Guild's name and operations echo the medieval trade associations and unions that regulated commerce and provided protection for merchants. The description of feudal trade implies that it is backward, creating the sense that society cannot move past the old ways. Overall, the balance of power between the three groups revolves around land, military forces, and economic profits.

Bound together in a feudal structure, these factions are dependent on one another. A change in fortunes for one creates ripple effects for the others. This is a universe with the rigid faufreluches class system, where everyone is kept in their place. It is not a world where people value or strive for equality. It also does not seem like a particularly science fictional world, aside from the concept of interstellar travel. The political set-up is historically based and familiar, requiring few details for us to grasp how it operates. Rather than spending time explaining a new political structure, Herbert maps his story onto pre-existing concepts so he can focus on the consequences to a change in the system.

There is another important faction that sits alongside the feudal order and operates more subtly: the Bene Gesserit. This all-female organization acts as a quasi-religious order that inserts itself at all levels of society by deploying women as wives, concubines, missionaries, and Truthsayers. It fulfills the historic role of the Catholic Church in not holding traditional monarchical positions yet still exerting significant influence on affairs of state as advisors, confessors, and leaders of religious and educational institutions.

Herbert also makes a crucial decision to remove advanced technology as a significant political factor by creating the backdrop of the Butlerian Jihad, "the crusade against computers, thinking machines, and conscious robots" [2, p. 521]. The Jihad represents a pivotal moment in the historical context of *Dune* because it put a halt to technological advancement and forced a focus on human development [5, p. 311, 313; 6]. The name signals an intertextual connection with Samuel Butler's satirical novel *Erewhon* (1872), in which mechanical inventions had been deemed too dangerous and were destroyed and their re-creation was forbidden. The context of the Jihad helps explain the existence of a feudal society in the future, but also narrows the scope of science fiction elements to enable Herbert to focus on humans rather than technology. It is additionally important for explaining the extreme importance of Arrakis and its spice melange: because humans need this substance to gain extraordinary abilities in the absence of advanced technology.

IMPERIALISM

With a feudal system making the lines of power visible, Herbert can more readily show us the corruptive nature of the imperialist and Machiavellian strategies of the groups jockeying for control. Through the characterization of the decadent and power-hungry Emperor and House Harkonnen, we can see the careless and exploitative nature of imperialism and colonialism.

As a key symbol of imperialism in *Dune*, the Emperor is associated with jealousy, treachery, and decadence. It is suggested he is greedy for profits from Combine Honnete Ober Advancer Mercantiles (CHOAM)—the universal development corporation controlled by himself and the Great Houses—and jealous of his own distant cousin Duke Leto's popularity among the Great Houses. His bargain with House Harkonnen to secretly provide Sardaukar troops to go after Leto signals his willingness to undermine the feudal order by betraying those who have pledged fealty to him. The vocabulary of decadence is used to show the Emperor's weakness as a ruler and link with classic portrayals of the decadent Byzantine court [7, p. 273; 8]. When he comes to Arrakis to see an end to the Harkonnen's mismanagement, he complains about having to delay or cancel court functions and affairs of the state. He brings a large entourage of "fringe parasites of the Court": pages, court lackeys, and women and their hairdressers and designers [2, p. 458]. Content with the five legions of Sardaukar he has brought, the Emperor has little understanding of the coup that Paul will soon initiate. He is also oblivious to the state of his troops. Weakened over time by overconfidence and cynicism, the Sardaukar find themselves overwhelmed by Fremen fighters, including women and children. Furthermore, the Emperor's compact with the Bene Gesserit has resulted in him having no legal sons, which places him in a vulnerable position in a society that prefers male succession. His line is poised to come to an end, to be replaced by Paul's, and the decadent Imperium is about to be overrun by the vigorous desert-dwelling Fremen population [7, p. 279]. Essentially, the Imperium is being disassembled by Paul and the Fremen, to be replaced by a new empire containing components of Fremen culture and military power, reflecting fourteenth-century historian Ibn Khaldun's theory that nomadic outsiders are well positioned to conquer wealthy urban civilizations due to their higher levels of solidarity and survival skills [9, p. 47, 49]. Yet the Emperor cannot envision a scenario in which he is not profiting from unlimited imperial wealth and encouraging the steady colonial extraction of spice on which his reign depends.

Meanwhile, the Harkonnen are portrayed as ruthless and selfish colonizers. Eighty years mining the spice on the fief of Arrakis to fulfill a CHOAM contract and enrich themselves is not enough to quell Harkonnen ambitions. The Harkonnen represent new money, having received their titles "out of the CHOAM pocketbook," and begrudge Leto's pedigree as the Emperor's cousin, however distant [2, p. 64]. They covet more than their present position, with the Baron aiming for his family to ascend to the imperial throne someday. Having stockpiled spice for twenty years, they have positioned themselves to benefit when Leto fails to meet the status quo level of spice production on his new fief. They are selfish rulers as well, and the few descriptions of their colonial regime are not flattering. Since the Harkonnen's only concern is spice, they make no pretense at being benevolent rulers or making improvements. Their system is full of bribery, and they spend as little as possible on providing for the local populace and outright hunt the Fremen for sport. Their approach to governance can be summed up with the Baron's instructions to his nephew Rabban: "You must squeeze [...] Don't waste the population, merely drive them into utter submission. You must be the carnivore, my boy" [2, pp. 239–240]. Their desire for more power and wealth drives them to inhumane behavior, suggesting that imperialist and colonial expansionism knows no bounds.

The Emperor and House Harkonnen's careless attitude toward the people under their rule and concern with power and profit above all else showcase their moral bankruptcy and unfitness to lead. Their embrace of imperialism and colonialism at all costs signals the corruptive nature of these systems. There are echoes of real-world colonialism, wherein Western nations established colonial outposts to expand their empires and gain access to valuable resources such as spices, jewels, and precious metals. Colonized peoples faced varying degrees of oppression and exploitation once their lands fell under imperialist control, and the legacies of colonial influence have remained long after the formal ending of colonial rule. Yet Herbert does not necessarily present decolonization as the answer, given that Paul keeps the structures of the Imperium, and the author hints that the Fremen might have been better working toward land rights and autonomy rather than seizing control of the government of their oppressors [10, p. 206].

There is also a clear parallel with economic imperialism in the Middle East. During the twentieth century, Western interest in the lands of the Middle East increased dramatically as oil became one of the most valuable resources. Backed by governmental support, Western businesses pursued contracts to secure a hold on petroleum reserves. Their concern was profit, not local populations or economies. In fact, there are several other elements that strengthen this connection in *Dune*: Arrakis as Iraq, spice as oil, and CHOAM as OPEC or other groups seeking to extract as much profit out of the sands as possible. When we examine the Emperor and House Harkonnen, we see they are driven by jealousy and a hunger for power, rather than the needs of their people. They view the Fremen disdainfully as barbarians or mongrels getting in their way. They even risk the political stability of the Imperium through their schemes on Arrakis [7, p. 278]. As the main representatives of imperial and colonial systems, the Emperor and House Harkonnen as villains signal the corruptive nature of these systems.

MACHIAVELLIANISM

However, if we see the Emperor and House Harkonnen as the bad guys and House Atreides as the good guys coming in to save the day, we have fallen for a trap that Herbert sets. There is more to this simplistic opposition of political factions than meets the eye. There are clues in *Dune* warning us that the Atreides have much in common with the Harkonnen, and in fact are just more effective at using Machiavellian strategies to maintain leadership and power.

Machiavellianism refers to a type of political philosophy based on the ideas of the sixteenth-century Italian political theorist and diplomat Niccolò Machiavelli. In his work *The Prince* (1532), Machiavelli explained how leaders could rule more effectively and advised that it was better to be feared than loved, and it was justifiable to be unscrupulous or amoral at times. His name came to be associated with political craftiness and the use of strategic manipulation, and the term Machiavellian is almost always a negative one, applied to characters or people who are cunning, manipulative, and power-hungry.

The Baron in particular represents an extreme version of the stereotypical Machiavellian villain, who enjoys evil and seeks to utterly destroy their enemies. Such a figure was popular in Elizabethan and Jacobean drama, exemplified by characters such as Shakespeare's Richard III and Iago [11, p. 26]. Their tools include betrayal, poison, and backstabbing, along with elaborately crafted plots that provide entertainment for the audience. Through the alternating perspective chapters in *Dune*, we see the Baron at work, gloating over his own craftiness. With the help of his Mentat, Piter de Vries, the Baron enacts a complex scheme to reclaim Arrakis, involving a traitor in the Atreides household, covert assistance from the Emperor, and a plan to use one nephew against the other. This plan to pressure Rabban into extracting large amounts of spice from Arrakis in a brutal regime, then to bring in Feyd-Rautha as a savior figure, can be found in Machiavelli's recounting of a similar scheme by Italian nobleman Cesare

Borgia in *The Prince* [11, p. 24–25]. We also see the Baron narrowly escape from the consequences of his plotting as his victims try but fail to take revenge (see Fig. 2.1). Overall, the Baron is a character who cares only for money and power, and without children of his own (to his knowledge) he schemes for himself and for his nephew in the hope of having the latter inherit the imperial throne.

On the other hand are the Atreides, the ostensible heroes of the story who possess everything the Harkonnen do not: self-control, honor, and respect for human life. Yet there is a disturbing similarity between the two [11, p. 25]. The Atreides also desire power and wealth for themselves and their noble house. Leto drags his family from their safe seat on Caladan to a dangerous desert planet at the bequest of the Emperor, but also in hopes of securing a larger fighting force and spice profits. Like the Baron, he

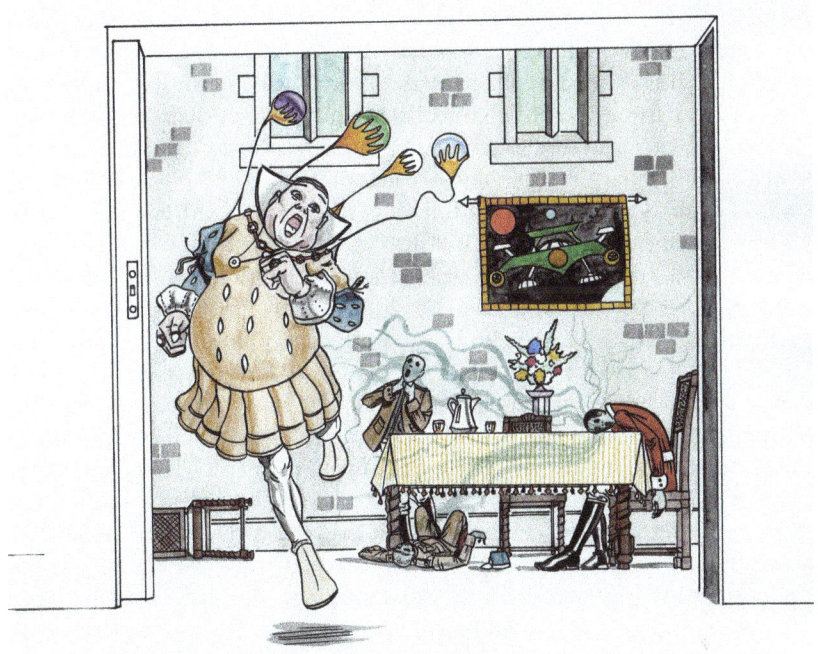

Fig. 2.1 Baron Vladimir Harkonnen fleeing from the poison released by his prisoner, Duke Leto Atreides. *Reproduced with permission from illustrator Arthur Whelan*

wants to see his family line continue to rule and is willing to do what is necessary to ensure this. Neither questions the colonizing of Arrakis or the manipulation of others to achieve their goals, whether that be the Emperor and his troops or the Fremen. Both the Baron and Paul also are good at planning surprises in order to win. The Baron succeeds in turning Dr. Wellington Yueh traitor, while Paul uses atomics on the Shield Wall and a sandworm attack to force the Emperor to abdicate. Ultimately, though they perish before seeing it, both the Baron and Leto get what they want: a male heir (via Jessica) who becomes a ruler.

If we see the Harkonnen as bad and the Atreides as good, we overlook how both arrogantly believe they are best suited to controlling everyone around them [12, p. 45]. Granted, the Atreides have more self-control than the Harkonnen, but nevertheless they use and abuse people as needed to secure power and authority. In revealing the plot twist that the Atreides actually share a kinship with the Harkonnen, Herbert further points us toward the idea that these are birds of the same feather. Leto dies before he is completely corrupted, but Paul is set to become the next tyrant who unleashes a destructive jihad, even as he masks his hunger for power under the guise of helping the Fremen [11, p. 30]. In comparing the two, we can arguably conclude that the Atreides are "the genuine followers of Machiavelli—the ones really to fear" [11, p. 28]. Herbert warned against falling for the admirable nature of the Atreides as part of his critique of the superhero: "But don't lose sight of the fact that House Atreides acts with the same arrogance toward 'common folk' as do their enemies. ... I am showing you the superhero syndrome and your own participation in it" [12, p. 45]. How effectively Herbert conveyed his message is up for debate, since so many readers see no reason not to celebrate Paul's rise to power, having spent the book identifying with his perspective and following him on his journey. Herbert's critique is largely unformulated, lying in pieces that we must put together to see the larger picture [13, p. 29]. But for those who notice it (or continue reading the series), the message is to beware those seeking after power, no matter how good or well-intentioned they may seem. Though we do not see the full cost of the looming jihad in *Dune*, noticing the similarities between the heroes and villains should prompt us to be more skeptical of whoever seems to be the 'good guys.'

Religion

Religion and religious manipulation are also significant features of the political landscape in *Dune*, for politics and religion go hand in hand. Herbert imagines that "elements of most ancient religions, including the Maometh Saari, Mahayana Christianity, Zensunni Catholicism and Buddislamic traditions" have been brought together in one scripture, called the Orange Catholic Bible [2, p. 525]. Yet this does not mean everyone has become a faithful follower of one religion or deity. Some rely on quotes from the O.C. Bible in times of crisis but do not worship a higher power, while others like the Fremen follow a mixture of their own religious beliefs and Bene Gesserit propaganda. The religious influences in *Dune* create a unique blend of terminology, traditions, and beliefs based on real-world religions and philosophies—including Catholicism, Islam, Buddhism, and Taoism—with this section focusing on elements from the first two. Together, religious elements help focus our attention on the complexities of human cultures and prompt us to consider how religion can serve as a powerful political tool.

Elements from Catholicism provide a solid religious context for the workings of the Bene Gesserit, whose organization highlights the nature of religious manipulation in action. The name and characterization of the Bene Gesserit point to them being like Jesuits and nuns, though without need of male oversight. They wear black hooded garments, take on titles such as Sister Superior and Reverend Mother, and value service and education. They essentially cloak themselves in the guise of religion as an effective way to operate with more secrecy and secure authority. Like the Jesuits, they engage in missionary activities to spread their reach. Through their Missionaria Protectiva, they sow various myths, including that a Bene Gesserit woman will arrive whose child will emerge as a savior figure with extraordinary powers. This messianic myth appears to be a stock-standard concept, something that is flexible enough to be used by anyone, which is part of what makes it so attractive yet dangerous. On Arrakis, Jessica soon discovers how deeply the Fremen absorbed the propaganda, even to the point of using the same terminology such as Reverend Mother. And Paul discovers that the people are already shouting the name Mahdi, referring to a messianic figure, at him when he rides through the streets of Arrakeen, recalling the image of Jesus being welcomed and praised on his way into Jerusalem by a crowd with palm branches.

This set-up enables Herbert to show religious manipulation as an added dimension of the Atreides' political ambition. Both Jessica and Paul quickly become entrapped by this religious web as they exploit the Fremen's beliefs. Jessica banters words with the Fremen housekeeper, the Shadout Mapes, which causes Mapes to believe Jessica is the one foretold in the legends and spread the word among the Fremen. As we see this explicit manipulation of Mapes' beliefs, we also see Jessica acknowledge that even she cannot help following this path: she wonders, "*Why do I play out this sham?* But the Bene Gesserit ways were devious and compelling" [2, p. 53]. After Paul impresses Liet-Kynes, the ecologist tells the Fremen to find the exiled child and protect him, essentially becoming a John the Baptist figure who paves the way for Paul to gain acceptance as the Fremen's messiah. Following in the footsteps of the Bene Gesserit, Paul has little choice but to grasp religion as a political tool to secure authority, even as it entraps him into the path that leads to the jihad. Herein lies a message about the power of religion to mold human thinking and cultures beyond any individual's capacity to control them, discussed further in Chap. 5.

Herbert develops a more complex picture of religion as a part of human culture in the Fremen, even as he criticizes their susceptibility to dogma, superstitions, and control by the imperialists. The Fremen's characterization and storyline have strong Islamic and Arabic influences. The use of terminology and cultural aspects from the Middle East is a significant component of Herbert's world-building efforts, and helps provide a real-world link and contextual depth to the characterization of the Fremen as a people. Many of the terms used by the Fremen are either taken directly from Arabic or are modified versions. The great sandworm is called Shai-hulud, a name based on Arabic words that may mean either 'immortal thing' or the "old man of eternity" [14, p. 102; 15, pp. 117–118]. Arabic terms that pre-date Islam are also used: for instance, the term for the sun, Al-Lat, comes from the name for a pre-Islamic Arabian deity, Al-lāt [15, p. 120]. References to the Fremen's messianic religion are terms associated with Islam, such as Muad'Dib, Shari-a, tahaddi al-bushan, and Sayaddin [14, p. 103, 105; 16, p. 39]. Muad'Dib means teacher and resembles Mahdi, meaning 'rightly guided one' and referring to a Muslim religious leader or messianic figure; Shari'a refers to religious law [14, p. 103, 105; 15, p. 114; 17, p. 182]. In the Twelver Shi'a sect of Islam, it is believed the Mahdi, or Hidden Imam, will return and bring the Day of Judgement to the world. Furthermore, the general plot outline of *Dune* is similar to the spread of Islam in the seventh century and the more recent rise of Arab power due to petroleum demand [17, p. 182]. There is also a connection with the nineteenth-century Islamic holy war against Russian imperialism in the Caucasus detailed by Lesley Blanch in *The Sabres of Paradise* (1960), from which Herbert borrowed terms such as kanly and kindjal as well as Naibs, the leaders of the Muslim tribesmen involved in the conflict [18]. "Appendix II: The Religion of Dune" contains a variety of references to Muslim histories, practices, and beliefs, including the Kitab al-Ibar, the title of fourteenth-century historian Ibn Khaldun's book; the Azhar Book, a likely reference to Al-Azhar University founded in 972; and a Muad'Dib proverb that seems to be a paraphrase of a Qur'anic verse [19]. In Herbert's vision of the future, religion has not gone away but remains a powerful motivating force for human beliefs and behavior. Yet the Fremen's openness to religion is what leaves them particularly vulnerable to manipulation by outsiders, first the Bene Gesserit and then the Atreides. Through them, we see the role religion can play as a catalyst for political movements.

The question is whether the Arabic and Islamic influences are used merely to create an exotic, romanticized backdrop for a thorough critique of religion. Indeed, there is disagreement as to how generously to interpret the depiction of the Fremen. One perspective is that the fact that the Fremen have been seeded with the myths and legends of the Bene Gesserit's Missionaria Protectiva indicates that they are gullible and open to religious exploitation. This can be viewed as perpetuating Orientalist stereotypes of Arabic peoples being "simple, easily manipulated, religious, fanatical, and in need of leadership, usually provided by the west" [17, p. 183]. The similarities between Paul and Lawrence of Arabia suggest that the Atreides are content to help the desert-dwellers as long as this also works toward the family's larger imperialist goals, and there are elements of a white savior narrative in Paul's appearance as the liberator of the Fremen [20; 21, p. 104]. The Atreides are depicted as politically savvy, and religion provides a handy mechanism for winning over a people they need as military allies. As readers, we see behind Jessica and Paul's façade to gain the Fremen's trust. Like them, we know the messianic myths have been artificially planted and they are not truly converting; they are just capitalizing on religion as an opportunity for survival.

However, we may also consider that Herbert's criticism is not necessarily related to one particular culture, per se, but related to the potential of any religion to be used as a political tool of indoctrination and exploitation. In this case, it is a Catholic-like group seeding religious myths to an Islamic-like people, and it is the hope for a messiah to save them from harsh living conditions that makes the Fremen susceptible to Jessica and Paul's influence. Their worship of the sandworm as Shai-hulud, for instance, is not presented in a negative light, but rather as a sign of their respect for their environment and the living creatures they share it with. Paul himself becomes trapped in the messianic myths surrounding him, just as he becomes trapped by his prescient visions. We see that his character does not seem to fully grasp the implications of his actions, such as when he labels the Fremen's religion as simple and practical and Jessica insists, "Nothing about religion is simple" [2, p. 383]. Jessica is fully aware of the power of religion as a tool of manipulation and myth-making, and that the Fremen are just one of many peoples who have been visited by the Bene Gesserit's missionaries. This points to a criticism broader than one focused on any specific religion out of the Middle East.

Another view is that the depiction of the Fremen and their culture is a welcome part of the science fiction genre. For some readers, especially those more familiar with the terms and cultural backgrounds on which the Fremen are based, the book takes on an additional layer of meaning that showcases a world of Arab Futurism, where Arab culture and language have survived and thrived to become part of the language of the world [22]. There is support for the idea that "Muslimness is embedded in its underlying structure and themes," and that Herbert appears interested in using science fiction to explore how Islamic traditions might have shifted over time and influenced the development of society alongside other religious traditions [19]. Numerous examples in the book show that Herbert was thoughtful in choosing and adapting terms from Arabic and from Islamic history, and he reshaped them as he saw fit to create the imaginary content of his new world and a rich intertextuality [15, pp. 109–110]. In addition, Herbert shows both Jessica and Paul becoming part of the Fremen, with their identities being fundamentally altered by their deeper understanding and embracing of this new culture [14, p. 106]. Paul takes on multiple new roles and names based on Arabic words—Muad'Dib, Usul, and Lisan al-Gaib; Jessica becomes a respected religious leader among the Fremen as a Reverend Mother and births a daughter she names Alia, a feminine Arabic name [14, p. 106; 15, p. 115]. Liet-Kynes, too, represents a hybrid figure with a foot in both camps who reveals his faith when he murmurs a prayer while passing over a sandworm. Even though these characters' intentions are not pure, they nonetheless adopt the

Fremen's rituals and ways of life. This suggests that the depiction of the Fremen and their religion in relation to the imperialists is nuanced and complex. Yet the warning remains of how susceptible people are to religious indoctrination, and how it can lead to disastrous results, such as the jihad that Paul foresees. The lure of the messiah who promises paradise is seductive, Herbert tells us, but needs to be examined critically.

POLITICAL SYSTEMS

Like Tolkien, Herbert used a feudal, medieval-type setting for his epic story, though the authors vary in the degree to which they critique the trappings of feudalism. Some consider *Dune* more akin to epic fantasy than science fiction due to this setting, numerous Gothic elements, and the lack of emphasis on technology. It has a familiar, historical feel to it, more so than a futuristic one. It leans on readers' general understanding of historical events and cultures to reflect on power and vehicles of power from a distance. At the time of publication, it offered a more fully fleshed-out political-historical canvas and impression of complexity than existed in science fiction [23, p. 341]. It continues to be a work against which other science fiction stories that tackle an expansive scope with large themes are measured [24, p. 113]. *Dune* was also part of a shift in science fiction away from optimism in science and technology and toward a more pessimistic view: that even with interstellar travel and various gadgets, humans were still susceptible to the same pressures that they had always faced. Progress was not inevitable. Humans might even decide to revolt against technology and revert to feudalism as a way to order their world.

Dune's treatment of power, politics, and religion remains relevant at a time when technological advancements abound while other parts of human societies stay relatively unchanged. The political ecosystem described in the book may at first seem far removed from the twenty-first century, but in fact can map onto present-day systems in nations and business. Consider organizational hierarchies, monopolies, coups, take-overs, corporate colonialism, and boardroom politics. When an upset in the balance occurs, the players shift in response, generally to secure their own claims to wealth and power. Although there have been declines in religious affiliation in certain countries, religion has not gone away and remains a powerful motivating force for human beliefs and behavior. Herbert's depiction of a complicated relationship between different cultures and the rise of religious fanaticism has only become more poignant, with a pressing need for more robust cross-cultural communication and inter-religious dialogue. Where other authors offer clear-cut portrayals of the enemy to be defeated, Herbert craftily sets up his hero to act more and more like the villain as they both seek more authority and power. He suggests that we cannot easily judge on the outside who is good or bad, and even the good guys can lead us astray. *Dune* shows us people's tendency to blindly follow leaders who promise to solve their problems, whether they come from a religious context or not. It challenges us to confront our own complicity in political and religious systems that we may be better guarded against their pitfalls in the real world.

References

1. Herbert, Frank and Beverly. Interview by Willis E. McNelly. 3 Feb. 1969.
2. Herbert, Frank. *Dune*. 1965. Berkley, 1984.
3. Daniels, Joseph M. *The Stars and Planets of Frank Herbert's* Dune*: A Gazetteer*. 1999.
4. Dunbar, M.J. "Greenland During and Since the Second World War." *International Journal*, vol. 5, no. 2, 1950, pp. 121-140.
5. DiTommaso, Lorenzo. "History and Historical Effect in Frank Herbert's 'Dune.'" *Science Fiction Studies*, vol. 19, no. 3, 1992, pp. 311-325.
6. Kennedy, Kara. "The Softer Side of *Dune*: The Impact of the Social Sciences on World-Building." *Exploring Imaginary Worlds: Essays on Media, Structure, and Subcreation*, edited by Mark J.P. Wolf, Routledge, 2020, pp. 159–174.
7. DiTommaso, Lorenzo. "The Articulation of Imperial Decadence and Decline in Epic Science Fiction." *Extrapolation*, vol. 48, no. 2, 2007, pp. 267–291.
8. Lau, Maximilian. "Frank Herbert's Byzantium: Medieval-Futurism and the Princess Historians Irulan and Anna Komnene." *Discovering* Dune: *Essays on Frank Herbert's Epic Saga*, edited by Dominic J. Nardi and N. Trevor Brierly, McFarland, forthcoming.
9. Rudd, Amanda. "Paul's Empire: Imperialism and Assemblage Theory in Frank Herbert's *Dune*." *MOSF Journal of Science Fiction*, vol. 1, no. 1, 2016, pp. 45–57.
10. Immerwahr, Daniel. "The Quileute *Dune*: Frank Herbert, Indigeneity, and Empire." *Journal of American Studies*, vol. 56, no. 2, 2022, pp. 191–216.
11. Mulcahy, Kevin. "The Prince on Arrakis: Frank Herbert's Dialogue with Machiavelli." *Extrapolation*, vol. 37, no. 1, 1996, pp. 22–36.
12. O'Reilly, Timothy. *Frank Herbert*. Frederick Ungar, 1981.
13. Touponce, William. *Frank Herbert*. Twayne Publishers, 1988.

14. Kennedy, Kara. "Epic World-Building: Names and Cultures in *Dune*." *Names*, vol. 64, no. 2, 2016, pp. 99–108.
15. Ryding, Karin Christina. "The Arabic of *Dune*: Language and Landscape." *Language in Place: Stylistic Perspectives on Landscape, Place and Environment*, edited by Daniela Francesca Virdis, Elisabetta Zurru, and Ernestine Lahey, John Benjamins Publishing Company, 2021, pp. 105–123.
16. Csicsery-Ronay, Jr, Istvan. *The Seven Beauties of Science Fiction*. Wesleyan University Press, 2008.
17. Zaki, Hoda M. "Orientalism in Science Fiction." *Food for Our Grandmothers: Writings by Arab-American and Arab-Canadian Feminists*, edited by Joanna Kadi, South End Press, 1994, pp. 181–187.
18. Collins, Will. "The Secret History of Dune." *Los Angeles Review of Books*, 16 Sept. 2017. https://lareviewofbooks.org/article/the-secret-history-of-dune
19. Durrani, Haris. "The Muslimness of *Dune*: A Close Reading of 'Appendix II: The Religion of Dune.'" *Tor.com*, 18 Oct. 2021. https://www.tor.com/2021/10/18/the-muslimness-of-dune-a-close-reading-of-appendix-ii-the-religion-of-dune/
20. Kennedy, Kara. "Lawrence of Arabia, Paul Atreides, and the Roots of Frank Herbert's Dune." *Tor.com*, 2 June 2021. https://www.tor.com/2021/06/02/lawrence-of-arabia-paul-atreides-and-the-roots-of-frank-herberts-dune/
21. Jacob, Frank. *The Orientalist Semiotics of* Dune: *Religious and Historical References within Frank Herbert's Universe*. Büchner-Verlag, 2022.
22. Ali, R. "Beside the Sand Dunes: Arab Futurism, Faith, and the Fremen of Dune." *Discovering* Dune: *Essays on Frank Herbert's Epic Saga*, edited by Dominic J. Nardi and N. Trevor Brierly, McFarland, forthcoming.
23. Roberts, Adam. *The History of Science Fiction*. 2nd ed., Palgrave Macmillan, 2016.
24. Riggs, Don. "Future and 'Progress' in Foundation and *Dune*." *Spectrum of the Fantastic: Selected Essays from the Sixth International Conference on the Fantastic in the Arts*, edited by Donald Palumbo, Greenwood Press, 1988, pp. 113–117.

CHAPTER 3

Ecology and the Environment

Abstract This chapter focuses on the depiction of the environment and people of the planet Arrakis, otherwise known as Dune. It explains the origins of Herbert's story in his research on the control of sand dunes in Oregon, and how the book tapped into the emerging movements of ecological awareness and environmentalism in the wake of ecologist Rachel Carson's revolutionary book *Silent Spring*. The chapter discusses the role of the ecologist, Dr. Liet-Kynes, in explaining scientific principles to readers even as he overlooks the consequences of his terraforming project and his trust in a hero figure. It recognizes the pivotal role of *Dune* in offering detailed world-building and an important environmental message about humans' disruption of ecosystems.

Keywords Science fiction • Frank Herbert • Ecology • Environment • Science • Terraforming

Dune is a novel born out of the natural environment. Dedicated to dryland ecologists, it invites us to see how everything is interconnected: humans, animals, plants, resources, and human-made structures of politics, religion, and economics. It is a story in which some characters live in harmony with nature and build their society accordingly, and others seek only to extract riches from the sand. And yet both sides are guilty of disrupting the desert planet's ecosystem toward selfish ends. In this chapter, we discuss the environment and people of the planet Dune. We explore the role of the ecologist in explaining scientific principles to readers even as he overlooks the adverse consequences of his terraforming project and his trust in a hero figure. We also examine Herbert's criticism of humans' desire to control and exploit nature rather than conserve it, which helps reveal the features that make *Dune* an influential work of ecological science fiction.

THE SCIENCE OF ECOLOGY

The science fictional basis and one of the primary themes of *Dune* is the science of ecology [1, p. 648; 2, p. 12]. According to Herbert, the idea for *Dune* originated in his research for an article about the control of sand dunes in Florence, Oregon, by the U.S. Forest Service, an agency under the U.S. Department of Agriculture [3, p. 102]. He became fascinated with the concept of controlling the dunes by treating them like waves. But he also saw beyond the seemingly simple outcome of changing a 'bad' situation of sand covering the highway to a 'good' situation. To him, the project linked with Western culture's tendency to inflict itself on the environment and view it as a collection of mechanical things that enough data could overcome and subdue. In this case, the government was finding great success in employing an ecological approach (planting grasses) instead of an engineering one (building a wall) [4, p. 39]. However, it was still seeking control of nature, order, and stability. From this starting point, Herbert drew together research on deserts, their peoples, and their religions, and created an entire planet of sand dunes where humans have adapted to the extreme environment but an ecologist seeks to transform it [4, p. 39].

In tapping into the emerging movements of ecological awareness and environmentalism, *Dune* helped popularize interest in humans' understanding of the natural world and their place in it, as well as their responsibility to conserve the precious resources it provided for them. Preceding it was ecologist Rachel Carson's revolutionary non-fiction book *Silent Spring* (1962). Carson sought to warn people about the threat to the balance of nature caused by poisonous pesticides, and her book "has continued to be a central text in the contemporary environmental movement worldwide" [5, p. 45]. It stands as a "fundamental social critique of a gospel of technological progress" and scientists' "irresolute carelessness of the natural world," themes which appear in *Dune* as well [6, p. 429]. In a sense, Carson's opening scene is science fictional—an imaginary town experiences "a strange blight" followed by sickness and death, and the twist is that the people have poisoned themselves [7, p. 2]. Like Carson, Herbert could write in a style that appealed to a popular audience. They both found a way to embed their messages about ecology and the environment through an insightful blend of storytelling and scientific ideas.

On this point, it should be noted that ecology is sometimes considered to be synonymous with the environment, but they are different terms. Ecology is the "study of the relationships between organisms and their environment" [8]. It recognizes the interconnectedness and interdependence of life. The environment refers to "the complex of physical, chemical, and biotic factors that act upon an organism or an ecological community and ultimately determine its form and survival" [9]. Ecological systems, or ecosystems, are created through the relationships between organisms and their environment. Feedback loops are an important feature of ecosystems. They occur when a change in one part of the system affects other parts, and then that change 'feeds back' to affect the original part. Feedback can be negative (balancing out the change and keeping the system in balance) or positive (intensifying the change and leading to greater change). For a basic example, if an animal population in an area increases, the animals will consume more food, but any predators of those animals will also have more food. The predators will then reduce the rate of the animal population increase and keep the system in balance. If there are no predators, though, the animal population will continue to increase until the food supply runs out. The terms 'ecology' and 'ecosystem' first appeared in the second half of the nineteenth century and experienced a sharp increase in usage between 1963 and 1973 [10]. This tracks with these topics' entrance into American literature and culture, in part due to the popularity of ecology-focused works such as *Silent Spring* and *Dune*.

Dune can be considered ecological science fiction for several reasons. It emphasizes the natural world through its focus on a desert environment and the adaptations humans and animals have made to survive there. It shows the interconnected webs of relationships of people and factions in the Imperium and the way everything centers on one resource. It also reveals the shifts in the balance of power as each faction struggles to gain more for itself, and the feedback loops that happen when a hero or messiah or scientist is introduced into an ecosystem. It is environmental science fiction because it offers a critique of the human tendency to control and exploit nature in an unsustainable way.

The Environment and People

Part of *Dune*'s staying power is that, decades after publication, the book still captures readers with its imaginative desert landscape. The planet Arrakis, or Dune, looms large as a place that is both known and unfamiliar, resembling the sandy landscapes of the Middle East but with fantastical, magnificent sandworms. We are introduced to Dune through the eyes of the fifteen-year-old Paul Atreides. Born into privilege and highly educated, Paul is curious about his family's move from the water-covered Caladan to the punishing climate of this desert wasteland. He asks his teachers about the people there, the lifestyles, and the reason they are going. His interest spurs ours. It sounds dangerous and intriguing. After his arrival, he continues piecing together various snippets of information, building up a picture in our minds of this new world before he has even set foot on the sand.

The endless desert with its shifting sand dunes is the dominant environmental feature of Dune, barren yet teeming with life in certain areas. By creating a world with one dominant ecosystem, as other science fiction writers have done, Herbert draws attention to the desert and the adaptations that life must make to survive in such a place. Most relate to moisture conservation. Whether native or introduced, the flora and fauna must adapt. Many of the birds live without water by drinking blood. The desert "climate demands a special attitude toward water. You are aware of water at all times. You waste nothing that contains moisture" [11, p. 113]. In a strange twist, the giant sandworms that stand out as the most memorable creatures find water poisonous. The Appendix implies that they were responsible for the formation of the deserts in the first place. Thus, the sandworms and the desert go hand in hand—these titans need the arid environment to produce the precious spice, melange, which is part of a circular relationship that involves little sandworms, pre-spice masses, fully developed sandworms, and sand plankton.

Spice also highlights the ecological principle of interconnectedness. It is a key feature of many other relationships in the Imperium and acts as a way for Herbert to tie together various threads in his world, including: "Fremen and the desert, the Great Houses and Arrakis, the Emperor and his throne, the Guild and interstellar travel, the Bene Gesserit and their abilities, and Paul Atreides and prescience" [12, p. 448]. Because everything is dependent on this one resource, we see the consequences when its supply is threatened or disrupted.

The environment is so prominent in the story that the planet Dune can be considered a protagonist in its own right [13, p. 16]. Not only is the novel named after it, but the active features of its desert help make it seem alive. Sandstorms roll in and force characters to fight their way through or wait them out. They disrupt communications equipment and cause heavy wear to other equipment such as spice mining machinery. Sandworms also represent an ever-present threat to anyone traveling through the open desert on foot. These exist in addition to the general heat and lack of water. The desert easily overrides human technology such as shields, lasguns, and communication devices. It demands that humans respond to it with caution and respect.

Though not originally from Dune, the Fremen are a people who have successfully adapted to and now live harmoniously within their environment. They provide a clear contrast to other groups that do not know or care about moving according to the rhythms of nature. Based on somewhat romanticized images of Native Americans, Bedouins, and other desert-dwelling populations, the Fremen survive on Dune by adhering to a strict 'water discipline' and working with the potential hazards rather than against them. They live in the coolness of caverns, and rest during the day and move in the dark. They have developed superior technology to conserve moisture, namely the stillsuits, and their bodies have ultrafast blood coagulation to reduce pointless moisture loss. They control and ride the sandworms using thumpers and hooks while harvesting the spice and using the poisoned water from drowned worms in their ceremonies and rituals. They also craft the infamous crysknife weapons from the sandworms' teeth. And they do not suffer outsiders but are fiercely loyal to their own. The Fremen are a strong and hardy people by necessity, and they function efficiently and safely in the desert except when being raided by outsiders such as the Harkonnen and Sardaukar.

The Ecologist

Part of how Herbert makes the environment and associated ideas about ecology understandable to readers is by providing a guide in the form of a planetary ecologist named Dr. Liet-Kynes. Kynes was originally set to be the novel's hero, a kind of ecological prophet [2, p. 13; 4, p. 44]. However, Herbert decided to make him a significant supporting character instead and avoid having readers think that the book had all the answers [2, p. 13]. Kynes is the Imperial Planetologist, tasked with following in the steps of his late father, Pardot Kynes, First Planetologist of Arrakis, and performing scientific research as a servant of the Emperor. Kynes is a man with conflicted loyalties, for he belongs to an educated class like Paul and is supposed to be following Imperial orders, yet he is also revered among the Fremen. In fact, he is Fremen, born of a Fremen mother and raised in their community. Kynes thus represents a bridge between the two worlds that Paul will soon inhabit, as well as a John the Baptist figure who paves the way for Paul's acceptance among the Fremen. As a scientist, Kynes is justified in explaining to other characters, and thus to us, the science behind how ecosystems work and remain in balance. And as a Fremen, he can impress upon others a respect for the ecosystem of Dune.

His dual roles help make Kynes believable as the mouthpiece of ecological principles throughout the first part of *Dune*. Through exchanges such as those in the dinner party scene—where we see the Atreides interacting with several key political players on their new planet—Herbert embeds important messages to develop our awareness about the interactions between living things. In a conversation about whether blood-drinking carrion-eating birds on Dune are cannibals, Paul remarks that a young organism can find its worst competition from its own kind because they are "eating from the same bowl"; Kynes endorses his understanding of this "rule of ecology," that the "struggle between life elements is the struggle for the free energy of a system" [11, p. 137]. This opens the way for Kynes to knock down another guest's derogatory comment about the Fremen drinking the blood of their dead. Actually, he explains, the truth is that the Fremen reclaim the water of their dead because it is so precious and the dead do not need it anymore. Here, Kynes serves as a vehicle for relaying information about both ecology and the Fremen's practices in an objective, scientific fashion. Through his eyes, practices that could be framed as repulsive or primitive gain scientific validation and acceptability to the new rulers, the Atreides, and by extension us. Paul's own understanding of ecology and his application of whole-systems thinking to human affairs also gain validation from Kynes: "Paul picks up the ecological 'charisma' by a kind of resonance in the mind of the reader" [4, p. 71].

Kynes also helps to highlight *Dune*'s critique of Western society's tendency to control and exploit nature rather than conserve it. On the surface, this criticism is about the colonizers and their treatment of Arrakis. The Harkonnen's interest in the planet is only to stockpile the spice and enrich themselves. They are brutal oppressors who do not care about anyone outside their immediate family and sometimes not even them. The Atreides are more honorable, but they also continue spice mining and hope to fortify their family's standing. Neither family questions the need to feed the Imperium's insatiable desire for this resource, regardless of the potential consequences of spice extraction on the environment or the locals. Kynes vocalizes disgust at the narrowmindedness of this obsession with the colonial extraction of spice. He tells Leto, "Arrakis could be an Eden if its rulers would look up from grubbing for spice!" and later says to Paul, "[T]he Imperium sends here only its trained hatchetmen, its seekers after the spice!" [11, p. 113, 222]. In fact, the Atreides not only seek to mine the spice, but presume to ask the Fremen to put their bodies on the line for them as fighters to help prop up their noble house. Regardless of the colonizer, the planet and the Fremen face disruption due to the demand for spice. For readers who make the comparison with oil and the Middle East, the critique of foreigners seeking to exploit the natural world to gain access to a precious resource takes on an added dimension. Some consider *Dune* one of the best allegorizations of U.S. energy policy and Middle East imperialism in the genre of science fiction [14, pp. 266–267]. Everything centers on spice, and Jessica and Paul generally only express care about the Fremen's interests when they align with their own. Seemingly no one in the novel wants to conserve the environment, for even Kynes and the Fremen are secretly working toward large-scale change.

The more subtle critique of Western culture is related to the science-driven terraforming project, which seems like the opposite of the exploitative colonial enterprise. Following in his father's footsteps, Kynes too sees the planet as a machine that can be reshaped to fit humankind's needs and the Fremen as the ecological tool to do so, guided by his scientific hand. When the Fremen are promised a paradise on Dune—"Open water and tall green plants and people walking freely without stillsuits"—they revere Kynes and his father as holy men and readily assist with the transformation process [11, p. 291]. Their planting of grasses to control the dunes may

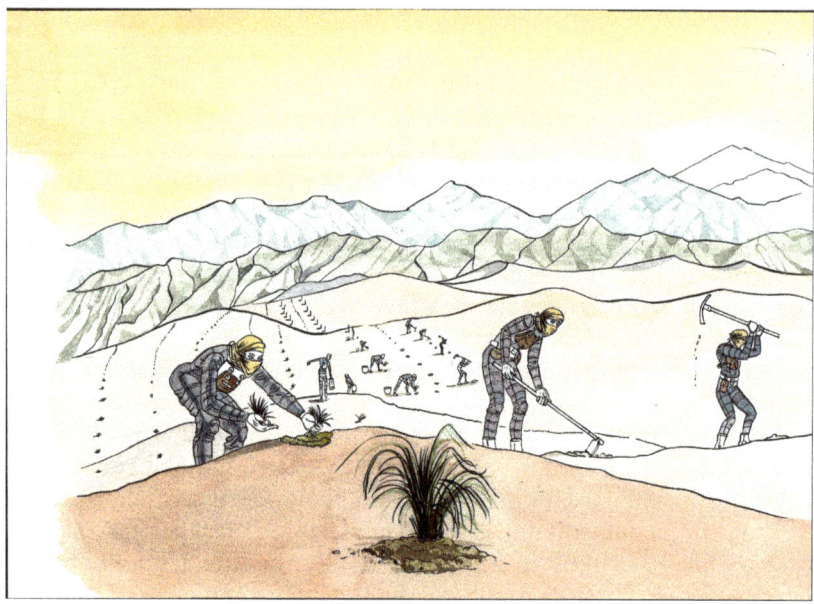

Fig. 3.1 Fremen planting grasses on dunes. *Reproduced with permission from illustrator Arthur Whelan*

remind us of the U.S. Forest Service's project in Oregon that sparked Herbert's interest in ecology (see Fig. 3.1).

But as with Paul, Kynes is a deceptively sympathetic character who may not appear malicious but can still initiate destructive forces. One feature that gives *Dune* its complexity is the use of such morally ambiguous characters who can prompt us to reconsider their motives. We want to believe that Kynes is doing good, that the Fremen's dream can come true. But if we do, we are placing too much faith in scientists who mistakenly think they have all the answers. Kynes' father rightly predicts that humans can alter the feedback systems and create a self-sustaining cycle to change the face of the planet. When he supposes that making a three percent change to the plants will start a cycle to transform the planet away from being an arid desert, he is viewing the ecosystem as one that can be radically changed if a key part of the system is shifted to cause a chain reaction [15, p. 56]. What both Pardot and Liet-Kynes fail to understand, however, is that despite knowing that "the highest function of ecology is the understanding of consequences," even an ecologist can never anticipate all of the consequences of such a project [11, p. 498].

Though both the scientists and the Fremen might seem to be working toward a positive end, the novel foreshadows that their disruption of the environment will have severe consequences for themselves and the universe. One sign revealed in the Appendix is that their first report on the plantings shows that sand plankton is being poisoned, poisonous water is forming that other lifeforms avoid, and a barren zone is spreading that even the sandworms will not invade. Pardot Kynes delights in this "gift from Arrakis" that has created a richer bed for plant life, but the terms "poisoned," "incompatibility," "poisonous," and "barren" sound ominous [11, p. 499]. Having just read that water is poisonous to the sandworms, and that they depend on sand plankton for food, we wonder how their survival will be managed. Then we learn that the sandworms are the main source of oxygen in the absence of plant cover, meaning that limiting their habitat may prompt an oxygen catastrophe [16, p. 354]. An even more obvious sign in the main storyline is the death of Liet-Kynes. Kynes' death in a spice blow after assisting Jessica and Paul serves as a warning against the idea that scientists have everything in hand. The image of Kynes is that of a person reduced to rags, without a stillsuit or water in the open desert. Yet still he serves as the voice of reason and explanation, as does his father, who appears to him in his delirium. But as Pardot drones on about their timetable of changing the planet, Liet has a sudden flash of clarity about a different future for Arrakis than his father had seen. We are left to wonder what this might be, and Kynes' final thought is that "his father and all the other scientists were wrong, that the most persistent principles of the universe were accident and error" [11, p. 277].

As Herbert and his spouse Beverly once discussed in an interview, Kynes' death is an important turning point that reveals one of the main purposes of the story: to show the "consequences of inflicting yourself upon a planet, upon your environment" [17]. Kynes represents a person from Western culture who has "lived out of rhythm" with the planet and as a consequence become swept up in its forces [17]. He is blinded by a belief that humanity can manipulate and control nature using data while somehow standing outside ecological processes. His parting thoughts thus suggest that it is false pride on the part of scientists to believe that they can fully understand the consequences of their actions and calmly separate themselves as creatures of the environment. This idea is echoed in the depiction of the Bene Gesserit, who also fail to control the outcome of their breeding program despite generations of planning. The death of the ecologist, the mouthpiece of science and reason, by a natural feature of the desert on Dune undercuts the idea that science has all of the answers, that enough data or technology can save humans from their destructive tampering. In its role as a protagonist, "[Liet-Kynes'] planet killed him" without care for his knowledge or intentions [11, p. 277]. Nature refused to be reduced to neat variables on a graph.

This undercutting of the scientist presents a cautionary message about the scientist's role in society. Rather than associating science with either the forces of the Imperium or the native peoples, Herbert offers a scientist character who belongs to both worlds yet still fails to grasp the nature of ecology. This places blame on both sides: the Imperium wants scientific knowledge about the planet since it is the only location of the precious spice, and the desert-dwelling Fremen want scientific knowledge to work toward making a more comfortable life for themselves. The message about science is ambiguous and asks that we consider its role in human affairs more carefully.

THE HERO

Herbert's critique of heroes runs as an undercurrent in *Dune*. This critique takes on an added ecological dimension through the characters of both Kynes and Paul as they leverage the terraforming project to gain control over the Fremen. Although they do not appear to have had much choice in their life path, neither turns away from the power his leadership position grants him. By following his father's lead, Kynes inflicts himself and his scientific vision onto the environment of Dune, drawing in others to follow him. The Fremen who once lived harmoniously with the desert and had adapted well now believe as the scientists do: that it is better to subdue nature and transform it to human desires. The Fremen revere Kynes so much that he eclipses tribal boundaries and is the only one who "speaks for all Fremen" [11, p. 283]. This status is essential to the story, for Kynes prepares the way for another heroic figure to swoop in and take advantage of the situation, directing followers on yet another path, that of the jihad that Paul foresees. Once Kynes decides to lend his support to Paul, this sets in motion a chain of events that will affect the planet and the entire universe. With Kynes gone, there is no one to challenge this course of action, this rapid acceleration of the project by a new hero; no one to speak the value of a slow, low-impact, natural evolution. Instead, the terraforming project is set to become an ecological disaster, spiraling beyond nature's ability to self-correct [4, p. 72]. With an increase in water and a retreating desert, it will be difficult to maintain a corner for the sandworms and spice. The great irony at the heart of *Dune* is that the ecologist actually helps set in motion the most significant disruption to the planetary ecosystem through leading the terraforming project and falling for the charisma of a young hero.

ECOLOGICAL SCIENCE FICTION

In creating this expansive desert ecosystem with its resilient local inhabitants, Herbert pioneered the development of detailed world-building in science fiction. Like Tolkien, he offered readers a world that is memorable and immersive, inviting them to return and experience it again. He also set the stage for an important environmental message: that we should be critical of the colonizers as well as the scientists who seek control at the expense of the planet and its people. They hold responsibility for the ecological disruptions that will transform not only the planet, but the universe.

Dune thus stands as a very influential ecological novel that has shaped not only popular culture but the treatment of ecology in the genre of science fiction [18, p. 118]. Though present in various ways previously, ecological awareness and themes were brought to the center of the genre by this book [19, p. 87]. It brought a holistic view of the role of humans in terraforming and linked the local with the global and nature with culture, though the full consequences of the terraforming project would not be seen until the sequels [18, pp. 118–120]. Other terraforming texts in the mid-twentieth century include Ursula K. Le Guin's *The Word for World Is Forest* (1972) and *The Dispossessed* (1974), which like *Dune* use planetary changes as a way to explore issues of politics and culture [18, p. 116]. Since these decades, ecological and environmental themes have come to form a more visible subgenre within science fiction. Notable texts include the *Mars* trilogy (1992–1996) by Kim Stanley Robinson, who acknowledged the influence of reading *Dune* as "an ecological primer on desert survival" [20, p. 253].

Dune does not offer us straightforward answers about how to live in balance with the environment and avoid ecological disaster. No person or group is perfect or fully understands their role in the bigger picture. What seems like a positive terraforming project includes a criticism of the desire to bend nature to human will regardless of the consequences. But the book does educate us about ecology and provide hints about what to avoid. It teaches us about the interconnectedness of living things and their environment, and how one change can have ripple effects in many directions. It suggests that a certain humility is needed when humans confront their place in the world. The Fremen have great respect for the sandworm and acknowledge their smallness in the face of the immense, moisture-starved desert they call home. Meanwhile, the colonizers see the sandworm as a dangerous beast that should be destroyed or avoided, and view the desert as a punishing wasteland that makes spice extraction costly. Although the ecologist respects the sandworms, he naively believes he can somehow relegate them to a corner of the planet and take the rest of the world for humans. We can map these viewpoints onto groups in our own world as we examine our relationship with the environment and how eager we are to shape it according to our selfish preferences rather than living in harmony with its rhythms. We can maintain skepticism when scientific or technological solutions are held out as a cure-all for a problem, especially when a charismatic personality is offering them. Perhaps most importantly, we can accept that no one is able to anticipate all of the consequences of a particular course of action, so we need to remain adaptable and open to change.

References

1. McNelly, Willis E. and Timothy O'Reilly. *"Dune." Survey of Science Fiction Literature*, vol. 2, edited by Frank N. Magill, Salem Press, 1979, pp. 647–658.
2. Touponce, William. *Frank Herbert.* Twayne Publishers, 1988.
3. Herbert, Frank. *Maker of Dune*, edited by Tim O'Reilly, Berkley Books, 1987.
4. O'Reilly, Timothy. *Frank Herbert.* Frederick Ungar, 1981.
5. Detweiler, Jane. "Rachel Carson, *Silent Spring* (1962)." *Literature and the Environment*, edited by George Hart and Scott Slovic, Greenwood Press, 2004, pp. 39–51.
6. Lear, Linda. *Rachel Carson: Witness for Nature.* Henry Holt and Company, 1997.
7. Carson, Rachel. *Silent Spring.* Houghton, 1962.
8. Smith, Robert Leo, and Stuart L. Pimm. "Ecology." *Encyclopedia Britannica*, 7 Feb. 2019. https://www.britannica.com/science/ecology
9. "Environment." *Encyclopedia Britannica*, 2 Jan. 2020. https://www.britannica.com/science/environment
10. GoogleBooks Ngram Viewer. https://books.google.com/ngrams/graph?content=ecology%2C+ecosystem&year_start=1860&year_end=2019&corpus=26

&smoothing=3&direct_url=t1%3B%2Cecology%3B%2Cc0%3B.t1%3B%2Cec
osystem%3B%2Cc0#t1%3B%2Cecology%3B%2Cc0%3B.t1%3B%2
Cecosystem%3B%2Cc0
11. Herbert, Frank. *Dune*. 1965. Berkley, 1984.
12. Kennedy, Kara. "Spice and Ecology in Herbert's *Dune*: Altering the Mind and the Planet." *Science Fiction Studies*, vol. 48, no. 3, 2021, pp. 444–461.
13. Kincaid, Paul. "The Great Dune Trilogy: A Review." *Vector*, 93 supplement, 1979, pp. 15–17.
14. Canavan, Gerry. "Of Further Interest." *Green Planets: Ecology and Science Fiction*, edited by Gerry Canavan and Kim Stanley Robinson, Wesleyan University Press, 2014, pp. 261–279.
15. Palumbo, Donald. "'Plots within Plots…Patterns within Patterns': Chaos-Theory Concepts and Structures in Frank Herbert's Dune Novels." *Journal of the Fantastic in the Arts*, vol. 8, no. 1, 1997, pp. 55–77.
16. McNelly, Willis E. "In Memoriam: Frank Herbert, 1920–1986." *Extrapolation*, vol. 27, no. 4, 1986, pp. 352–355.
17. Herbert, Frank and Beverly. Interview by Willis E. McNelly. 3 Feb. 1969.
18. Pak, Chris. *Terraforming: Ecopolitical Transformations and Environmentalism in Science Fiction*. Liverpool University Press, 2016.
19. Latham, Rob. "Biotic Invasions: Ecological Imperialism in New Wave Science Fiction." *Green Planets: Ecology and Science Fiction*, edited by Gerry Canavan and Kim Stanley Robinson, Wesleyan University Press, 2014, pp. 77–95.
20. Canavan, Gerry, and Kim Stanley Robinson. "Afterword: Still, I'm Reluctant to Call This Pessimism." *Green Planets: Ecology and Science Fiction*, edited by Gerry Canavan and Kim Stanley Robinson, Wesleyan University Press, 2014, pp. 243–260.

CHAPTER 4

Mind and Consciousness

Abstract This chapter discusses how *Dune* was groundbreaking in terms of its characters not because it gave them superhuman abilities, but because it made them three-dimensional and focused on the power of their minds. It looks at Herbert's intense interest in the nature of human consciousness and his use of different narration styles to make characters seem like real people struggling to survive on an alien planet. The chapter examines the complexity of the characterization of the Bene Gesserit with their extraordinary abilities based on Eastern philosophical traditions such as Zen Buddhism and Yoga. It also explores Paul Atreides as a superhuman figure who takes the reader on his journey of expanding awareness and points to the possibilities of the human mind.

Keywords Science fiction • Frank Herbert • Consciousness • Psychology • Mind • Eastern philosophy

Dune was not unique in science fiction for giving characters superhuman abilities or the status of a messiah. Nor was it special for using the archetype of the hero or including a psychoactive drug. What made it groundbreaking was the three-dimensional nature of its characters and its intensive attention to the power of the human mind. The hero and his mother seem like real people with a range of motivations, struggles, and emotional complexities. There is also a strong dose of Eastern philosophies that show alternative ways of thinking and being. In this chapter, we explore *Dune*'s focus on the human mind and consciousness. We look at how this connects with the development of complex characters with psychological depth who pull us into the world. We also examine the enhanced abilities of key characters and how these prompt us to consider the potential in altered states of awareness.

Characterization

Some might consider Herbert obsessed with the nature of human consciousness [1, p. 29]. It is infused throughout *Dune* and is one of the novel's major strengths [2, p. 653]. Herbert gives us characters who are "incredibly awake" and do not let life pass them by [2, p. 653]. He carefully sets up his main character to be hyperaware from the moment we meet him. Things do not just happen to Paul—he notes them, evaluates them, and responds to them [3, p. 63]. We gain access to his mental processes as his awareness expands, and we learn that his mother's Bene Gesserit lessons are part of why he behaves as he does. Although certain readers may find the first scene overwhelming due to the amount of detail, this opening is very significant: "Everything is in capsule, evocative, a seed for later pearls to crust upon" [2, p. 653].

To keep pace with such characters, we need to pay attention, to be aware ourselves. The entire book can be seen as an attempt by Herbert to broaden the consciousness of his readers under the pretense of following a hero's journey. Herbert is like a Zen master, asking us to question our assumptions and logical habits [4, p. 10; 5]. Readers are likely to feel their own consciousness expanding, as they not only learn about new objects such as ornithopters and stillsuits but also understand more about the awareness of characters such as Jessica and Paul [4, p. 24]. Jessica and Paul frequently showcase their ability to be hyperaware. Even though we see that they are not always in control and that their awareness has flaws, it bestows a kind of god-like status on them as they move through the world. And because the heightened awareness that characters experience is grounded in real perceptive abilities, we may feel that we could also achieve them, rather than write them off as fantastical [2, p. 654].

One way Herbert makes this all possible is by merging the usual pattern of a third-person narrator telling the story with a first-person inner perspective, making us feel like we are participating in events from the inside [2, p. 654]. He develops characters' thoughts and feelings in a complex way by layering the narrator's viewpoint alongside certain characters' internal thoughts and other characters' dialogue [4, p. 19]. The opening chapter sets the precedent for this technique. The narrator describes an old woman and the mother of a boy looking in on him in his bed and having a brief conversation about him. As soon as the narrator indicates the women have gone, we move to the boy's perspective: "Paul lay awake wondering: *What's a gom jabbar?*" [6, p. 4]. The italicization signals our direct access to his in-the-moment thoughts. And this leads us to identify with his perspective, since we too are wondering what the gom jabbar is. For the next few paragraphs, the narrator's description of Paul is interrupted by these italicized thoughts, which reinforce the sense that Paul is carefully considering his circumstances before his family's move to a new planet. We feel that we know this character better because we can see his mental processing. His thoughts show an uncertainty and vulnerability that make him seem relatably human.

This technique is subsequently used with the two women in this chapter—Lady Jessica and Reverend Mother Gaius Helen Mohiam—and then other characters throughout the book. It slows down the action, focusing our attention on how characters perceive and respond to their world. The dinner party scene gives us a prime example of Paul and Jessica's hyperawareness in the presence of other characters. Their Bene Gesserit skills in perception make them aware of and able to read a significant degree of body language. They constantly scan their environment and the people in it, analyzing important details rather than just existing in the moment. In this scene, the book goes back and forth on showing us the narrator's descriptions of Paul and Jessica's behavior, the characters' thoughts as they play the game of politics at the table, and their dialogue with their guests [4, p. 23]. We cannot help but see how much insight they gain. Certainly, other characters are also aware of how to play politics, but we gravitate to admiring Jessica and Paul's skills because we are seeing the scene play out through their consciousness. Each time we see Jessica and Paul perceiving and analyzing their environment, this adds to the sense of how important it is to be consciously aware.

Seeing how characters process the events in their lives adds layers of psychological depth to their personas. It builds out from their archetypal bases to make them more multi-dimensional. Paul is more than a stereotypical hero—he seems like a young man who is both eager to make his mark on the world and concerned about his future. Jessica is more than a stereotypical mother—she seems like a woman with conflicted feelings about the decisions she has made for her son and what will happen to her family. Through his characterization techniques, Herbert gives the illusion of psychological interiority, that characters are real people who think and feel just as we do. By inviting us to identify with Paul and Jessica, the narrative takes us along on their journey of awareness. Having access to their internal consciousness is essential to giving them a three-dimensionality and humanness that make them interesting and memorable.

Human Potential

Unlike science fiction stories that explore the nature of consciousness through non-humans such as robots or androids, *Dune* looks at it through different groups and training methods that expand human awareness. These include the Bene Gesserit, Spacing Guild, and Mentats, each of which has mastered its own specialization. The reason given for the focus on the human mind is the Butlerian Jihad, the ancient crusade against advanced technology that forced humans to develop themselves rather than rely on thinking machines. Herbert uses these groups to explore human potential and add meaning and depth to his characters and their abilities. He has both of his main characters receive training in the Way of the Bene Gesserit. Thus, Jessica and Paul have gained their enhanced awareness not on their own, but through the group most concerned with the power of the human mind and consciousness.

The Bene Gesserit

Herbert draws on multiple influences in his creation of the Bene Gesserit, giving the order a richness and complexity not found in the other groups. In addition to Catholicism, discussed in Chap. 2, another important influence comes from Eastern philosophies about the mind and body and altered states of consciousness, which contrast with those in a Western framework. In the Western philosophical tradition, the mind and body are considered separate things, a legacy of philosopher René Descartes' theory about a mind–body split. The mind is often seen to be superior to the body since it does the thinking and rationalizing. Descartes' famous statement "I think, therefore I am" refers to the idea that thinking is how we know we exist, so the mind is important as the source of our consciousness. But this view downplays the role the body plays in our existence in the world. It prioritizes conscious thought and reason and skirts over the fact that we often act without thinking and let our bodily needs and desires guide our behavior. Experiences or states of consciousness which do not have rational explanations or fit into neat boxes may be dismissed or mocked, including out-of-body experiences, drug trips, hypnosis, and dream states.

In contrast, Eastern philosophies have tended to have a more holistic view of mind and body that understands them as intertwined and mutually important. For instance, in Indian philosophy, the interconnectedness of mind and body can be considered a way of obtaining knowledge, with the mind actively involved in obtaining and coordinating the body's perceptions and sensations [7, p. 83]. In fact, some Indian philosophical traditions consider the human body to be a continuum that includes various physical and psychic components, which avoids the mind–body problem [8, p. 347]. Eastern civilizations have also given more acknowledgment and validity to altered states of consciousness in their religions and cultures [9, p. 139]. Traditions such as Yoga, Vedanta, and Buddhism, particularly Theravada, Mahayana, Vajrayana, and Zen Buddhism, emphasize the use of meditation and recognize different levels of mind and higher states of consciousness [9, p. 139]. Meditation becomes the basis for a state of enlightenment, and corresponding reductions in metabolic activity and even a suspension of breathing [9, p. 141]. In the U.S., the 1950s marked the beginning of a trend toward widespread awareness of Buddhism, Hinduism, and other Asian spiritual traditions, helped along by cultural shifts and the mass media [10, p. 4]. Zen Buddhism, in particular, gained notoriety in large part to the efforts of Japanese scholar D.T. Suzuki and his impact on influential figures such as the Beat poets and Alan Watts. Translated into Western culture, Eastern philosophies and associated practices such as Zen meditation and Yoga were valued as an alternative to Western rationality that could potentially help restore balance to a troubled modern world [10, p. 55].

Believing in self-development in a Zen sense himself, Herbert tapped into this emerging wave of interest in Eastern philosophies, as interpreted in the West, to give the Bene Gesserit a depth that makes the order and its abilities seem more realistic. Through the Bene Gesserit Way, they embrace a more holistic view of the mind and body and instill the kind of discipline that allows them to be more aware and in control. Their prana-bindu training lets them control their breath and survive an incredible expansion of consciousness through the spice drug ritual, detailed below. Indeed, the terms prana and bindu are Sanskrit and link with Indian notions of breath and meditation [11, p. 39]. The Bene Gesserit certainly see the benefits in accessing and understanding layers of consciousness beyond the ordinary. Despite their skills seeming almost magical to uninformed outsiders, some are very similar to what seasoned practitioners in the real world have mastered throughout history. *Dune* thus draws on beliefs about consciousness held by various peoples and cultures to enrich its character development.

The Bene Gesserit's preoccupation with the mind and consciousness is shown through their test of humanness, training regimen, use of the Voice, and access to Other Memory. The Bene Gesserit are the ones in the book most visibly concerned with what makes someone human, which they define as a person's ability to control their animal instincts. When Reverend Mother Mohiam has Paul put his hand into her black box and holds the poisonous gom jabbar needle at his neck, this tests Paul's ability to override his instinctual urge to pull his hand out and instead endure the painful sensations. Reverend Mother Mohiam casually tells Paul that a human can override any nerve in the body, as if it were a sensation that could easily be turned off when needed. The test of humanness prompts us to think about humans more deeply: What differentiates us from animals, if anything? How much control do we have over our nervous system? Would we be able to withstand the pain and pass the test? In the Bene Gesserit's eyes, a human must have a certain level of conscious control over their behavior, lest they fall prey to thinking machines again.

The Bene Gesserit have, therefore, developed a comprehensive training regimen to help people rise above their base instincts and live in a state of higher awareness. Such training is specifically designed to foster a high level of control over mind and body. The first hint at Bene Gesserit training we see is when Paul clears his tensions by practicing one of Jessica's mind–body lessons and finding "focused consciousness by choice" [6, p. 5]. As the story continues, we discover Jessica and Paul are extremely perceptive and can pick up on the smallest details in their environment. Prana-bindu training gives them complete control over their body's muscles (prana-musculature) and nerves (bindu-nervature). With this training, Jessica can control pregnancy and put herself into a hibernative state by stilling her breath, and both she and Paul can fight and win in unarmed combat. Another Bene Gesserit, Lady Margot Fenring, discusses how she plans to plant prana-bindu phrases in the unconscious mind of Feyd-Rautha Harkonnen in case he needs to be controlled at a future date. All of these abilities show how the Bene Gesserit have harnessed the power of the mind and body to be more fully aware and in control as they move through the world.

They also teach the Litany against Fear as a way of calming the mind in times of distress or peril: "*I must not fear. Fear is the mind-killer. Fear is the little-death that brings total obliteration. I will face my fear*" [6, p. 8]. Paul recalls the litany as he faces the test of humanness and the fight with Jamis, Jessica and Paul rely on it when caught in the 700–800-kilometer-per-hour winds while flying the ornithopter, and Jessica uses it when undergoing the dangerous Water of Life ceremony. The litany represents a type of prayer or mantra that helps the Bene Gesserit overcome a potentially overwhelming emotional response. It is a useful tool in their arsenal of conscious control that prevents them from acting on instinct.

Another ability of the Bene Gesserit, the Voice, highlights how they can control others at a level below conscious awareness. They understand that people often act without thinking and capitalize on this knowledge. When a Bene Gesserit uses the Voice, she adapts the tone and pitch of her voice to speak to someone in a way that compels them to obey. Reverend Mother Mohiam uses the Voice on Paul to command him to come near her for the test of humanness, though he is aware of the technique since he has been trained by his mother. Jessica uses it on Thufir Hawat to show him a glimpse of her extraordinary abilities. Once Paul has mastered it, he uses it several times, including on Reverend Mother Mohiam to show how his skills have matured beyond hers. The Voice reveals how easily some people can be led into behaving without consciously thinking about their actions [3, p. 47]. It reminds us that we may not be as rational and thoughtful as we have been led to believe.

Through the process of ingesting and neutralizing a large dose of the spice drug, the Bene Gesserit are able to enlarge their consciousness to include their ancestors' memories. This draws our attention to the limits and possibilities of expanding the human mind, as well as the capacity to experience events through someone else's perspective. Jessica's experience during the Water of Life ceremony shows us a brilliant example of human consciousness dying, expanding, and awakening. With the aid of the spice drug, the dying Fremen Reverend Mother Ramallo pours her memories into Jessica as her physical body collapses. Because the book gives us a look at the process from the inside, as the two women dialogue and Jessica describes her experience, we see Jessica's consciousness transformed—we know she has changed. In fact, we get more detail of Jessica's experience than of Paul's when he later takes the Water of Life, even though he is the one on the hero's journey. There is also a birth of consciousness when the fetus Jessica is carrying, the future Alia Atreides, is awakened to awareness. It is only later that we see the consequences of this procedure: Alia may have the body of a child, but her mind is that of an adult who is also already a Reverend Mother. The fact that she never had time to develop her own personality and consciousness haunts her later in life.

There are parallels here with Carl Jung's concept of the collective unconscious, but Herbert makes these ideas more concrete [4, p. 10]. Jung describes the collective unconscious as the part of the human psyche that is universal, impersonal, and identical in all individuals [12, p. 43]. In contrast to the personal unconscious, which develops uniquely in each person, the collective unconscious is inherited and made up of pre-existing forms that Jung calls archetypes. Although the Bene Gesserit's form of ancestral memory does not identically match this concept, it shares the notion that parts of the psyche can be inherited or passed down, either through a special ceremony or through the genes. Jessica's memory transfer heightens our awareness of things such as history, traditions, and rituals, and how individuals become a people and a culture. It also suggests that a person's consciousness can live on past death, in this case by hitching a ride in another person's mind.

Through the depiction of the extraordinary abilities of the Bene Gesserit, *Dune* embraces a more expansive view of consciousness and human potential. We learn about what it might look like if humans had a much higher level of conscious control over the mind and body and used it to their advantage, and the role of drugs in this process. But in Herbert's borrowing from various non-Western traditions, there is the possibility that these threads become a problematic way of exoticizing the story or characters. Other science fiction authors including Philip K. Dick and Ursula K. Le Guin used Eastern elements for the purpose of critiquing Western concepts of reality and progress [13, p. 25]. The line between cultural appropriation and respectful borrowing is debatable, particularly when Eastern traditions are dehistoricized and placed in front of readers who may have little to no understanding of their sources. The Bene Gesserit do have a mystical feeling about them, which serves the purpose of making the order mysterious and different from other groups. Words such as the Way and prana-bindu are based on Taoist, Buddhist, and Sanskrit terms and lend an exotic flavor to the order. The Bene Gesserit are also feared by others, some of whom label them as witches because of their powerful abilities. However, on the whole, the Eastern philosophies underpinning their order appear to be used cautiously and respectfully to help speculate on human potential. A key component of the Bene Gesserit's influence and success is their willingness to embrace a more holistic understanding of the human. This is a credit to the positive value of Eastern philosophies. The superhuman figure of Paul embraces a greater balance on his hero's journey, rather than rejecting it, which provides additional credibility to the potential in non-Western ways of thinking.

Guild Navigators, Mentats, and Suk Physicians

Although other groups are not developed with the same level of detail as the Bene Gesserit, their specialties also focus our attention on the power of the human mind. Not much detail is given about the Spacing Guild or its secretive navigators, but they too have pushed their limits and achieved a higher level of consciousness with the aid of the spice drug. They have a form of prescience that they use to safely guide spaceships through space, enabling them to maintain their monopoly on interstellar transport. Mentats take the place of computers in the *Dune* universe and are trained to assemble bits of logic and information to make predictions and perform calculations. They are very much focused on the mind and its ability to process data. Although this makes them vulnerable to faulty data and errors in their computations, they are considered useful for their projections of logic. The Suk Medical School produces physicians who undergo Imperial Conditioning to prevent them from harming patients, presumably making them trustworthy enough for the highest nobility. However, the Atreides' physician, Dr. Wellington Yueh, manages to overcome his conditioning and betray the family in his attempt to discover the fate of his Bene Gesserit spouse, Wanna Marcus, who has been tortured by the Harkonnen. Yueh's traitorous act emphasizes the ability of the conscious mind to go against previous training, and that there are no certainties if there is a powerful enough reason pushing someone to act. The characterization of these groups, while limited, reinforces *Dune*'s concern with the mind and its capabilities, showing how humans have attempted to fill the gap left by the banning of advanced technology.

Paul, the Superhuman

Paul's skillset goes beyond that of other groups—namely the Bene Gesserit, Guild, and Mentats—because his character combines their abilities into one person. As the protagonist of *Dune*, he takes us on his journey of expanding awareness and showcases different aspects of the human mind and consciousness along the way.

Paul's unique experience of consciousness is specifically linked with his genes. He represents the culmination of the Bene Gesserit's ninety-generation-long breeding program to produce the Kwisatz Haderach, a figure who can bridge space and time and tap into male ancestral memory as well as visions of the future. His consciousness is therefore genetically primed to expand beyond that of normal humans, and even of the women of the Bene Gesserit. As a hero figure, he is special, a person to watch as he matures into his destiny. However, rather than being a superhuman who magically stumbles upon extraordinary abilities, he has to grow them by undergoing rigorous training [14, p. 67]. We see brief glimpses of his training with his mother and his tutors, and can imagine how much effort has gone into molding this young man. This helps provide depth and believability to his character. His obsession with his growing abilities interests us and keeps pointing our attention to the nature of human consciousness and how it becomes expanded but also distorted in his person.

Paul's expansion of consciousness is also inextricably linked with spice, which is one of the most memorable substances in science fiction. Herbert's creation of spice as a type of psychedelic allows him to explore the possibilities of the human mind in a realistic way. Although spice is fictional, it has several connections to real-world drugs that help make its effects familiar and meaningful to readers [15]. Dreams usually remain confined to the unconscious realm, but in *Dune*, they break into Paul's waking consciousness as he matures and ingests higher concentrations of spice, which is produced as part of the lifecycle of the giant sandworm (see Fig. 4.1). Each time Paul dreams or envisions something, it reminds us of the power of the mind. It interrupts the action, letting us watch a person contemplate and consider, rather than impulsively act. Paul's drive to not be left in the dark about the future makes him seek more and more awareness and eventually more of the spice drug. Spice opens up new mental pathways for Paul, and he gains a greater understanding of himself. For instance, he discovers his Harkonnen heritage, which undermines his identity as an Atreides. Without a substance such as spice, Paul's

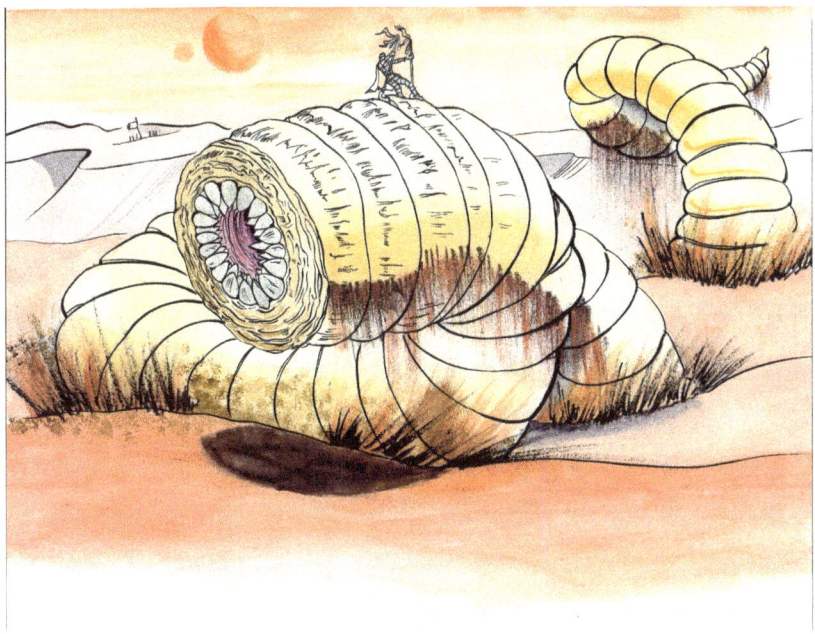

Fig. 4.1 Fremen riding the giant sandworm using maker hooks. *Reproduced with permission from illustrator Arthur Whelan*

experiences and visions might appear to be the workings of a madman. Having a prominent drug in the story helps make his abilities seem like a speculation on higher mental states of awareness, and helps keep us as readers focused on the possibilities of the human mind.

However, Herbert includes a warning that there can be such a thing as too much consciousness or awareness of the past and future. If we pay attention, we see that as Paul's awareness expands and he embraces the full extent of his special abilities, his humanity contracts. He begins losing touch with his emotions and his family's values, such as having a concern for human life. His young son's death seems to have no impact on him, and he expresses more concern for lost equipment than lost troop lives. He moves into a distant space, trapped to follow the path of his visions and his need for control and power. We as readers cannot identify with him to the same extent as we could at the beginning of the book. The expansion of consciousness has clear consequences for his character and suggests there is a cost to his superhuman abilities.

SOFT SCIENCE FICTION

Dune played a critical role in proving to readers beyond science fiction fans that a novel could be both science fiction and literature. At a time when the science fiction genre was struggling to move beyond underdeveloped or stereotypical characters and cliched scientific and technological inventions, *Dune* appeared as a lengthy book with multiple layers of complexity and thematic depth. It featured three-dimensional male and female characters who were interesting and memorable. It lived up to the growing expectation that writers should try to raise the literary and stylistic quality of science fiction [16, p. 335]. As one of the first science fiction bestsellers alongside Robert Heinlein's *Stranger in a Strange Land* (1961), *Dune* also proved that a story focused on the so-called soft sciences such as psychology, perception, and linguistics could be very successful [17]. Like other stories emerging in the 1960s as part of the New Wave of science fiction, *Dune* was concerned more with 'inner space,' the realm of the human mind and psychological concerns, than outer space, the domain of spaceships and technologies. This focus enabled Herbert to flesh out his characters and examine different aspects of consciousness, something that has long been of interest to humanity.

The book's focus on human potential is certainly an important reason for its success and has prevented it from becoming outdated. Interest in psychology has only increased since the 1960s. There are now many sub-branches of scientists who study the human mind, which in many ways remains a mystery, and many people are eager to study this topic to learn more about themselves and others. *Dune* raises the notion that there is much more to explore and understand about human consciousness than what rational-focused Western science has found so far. The popularity of yoga, mindfulness, and meditation signals a shift in Western culture toward a desire to create a more harmonious relationship between mind and body. This is complemented by a growing awareness and respect for the role the mind plays in overall wellbeing. In addition, although *Dune* does not offer a wholesale endorsement of drugs, it does suggest that there can be benefits to their ability to change human awareness. This idea is being validated with new waves of trials with psychoactive substances such as psilocybin and LSD for therapeutic treatment. It is likely that humans will always be fascinated by themselves and how they think and behave, so this places *Dune* in a good position to continue to influence readers for generations to come.

REFERENCES

1. Miller, David. *Frank Herbert*. Starmont House, 1980.
2. McNelly, Willis E., and Timothy O'Reilly. "*Dune.*" *Survey of Science Fiction Literature*, vol. 2, edited by Frank N. Magill, Salem Press, 1979, pp. 647–658.
3. O'Reilly, Timothy. *Frank Herbert*. Frederick Ungar, 1981.
4. Touponce, William. *Frank Herbert*. Twayne Publishers, 1988.
5. Smith, Tara B.M. "The Tangled Bank and the Ox's Tail: Reading *Dune* as a Zen Koan." 2017. University of Sydney, BA Honours Thesis.
6. Herbert, Frank. *Dune*. 1965. Berkley, 1984.
7. Chennakesavan, Sarasvati. *The Concept of Mind in Indian Philosophy*. Asia Publishing House, 1960.
8. Holdrege, Barbara A. "Body Connections: Hindu Discourses of the Body and the Study of Religion." *International Journal of Hindu Studies*, vol. 2, no. 3, 1998, pp. 341–386.
9. Shear, Jonathan. "Eastern Approaches to Altered States of Consciousness." *Altering Consciousness: Multidisciplinary Perspectives*, edited by Etzel Cardeña and Michael J. Winkelman, ABC-CLIO, 2011, pp. 139–158.
10. Iwamura, Jane. *Virtual Orientalism: Asian Religions and American Popular Culture*. Oxford University Press, 2011.
11. Kennedy, Kara. *Women's Agency in the* Dune *Universe: Tracing Women's Liberation through Science Fiction*. Palgrave Macmillan, 2021.
12. Jung, Carl. *The Archetypes and the Collective Unconscious*. Pantheon Books, 1959.
13. Huang, Betsy. "Premodern Orientalist Science Fictions." *MELUS*, vol. 33, no. 4, 2008, pp. 23–43.
14. Prieto-Pablos, Juan A. "The Ambivalent Hero of Contemporary Fantasy and Science Fiction." *Extrapolation*, vol. 32, no. 1, 1991, pp. 64–80.
15. Kennedy, Kara. "Spice and Ecology in Herbert's *Dune*: Altering the Mind and the Planet." *Science Fiction Studies*, vol. 48, no. 3, 2021, pp. 444–461.
16. Roberts, Adam. *The History of Science Fiction*. 2nd ed., Palgrave Macmillan, 2016.
17. Kennedy, Kara. "The Softer Side of *Dune*: The Impact of the Social Sciences on World-Building." *Exploring Imaginary Worlds: Essays on Media, Structure, and Subcreation*, edited by Mark J.P. Wolf, Routledge, 2020, pp. 159–174.

CHAPTER 5

Heroes and Masculinity

Abstract This chapter explores the complexity of the protagonist Paul Atreides and the ways he does and does not align with the hero archetype and stereotypical characteristics of masculinity. It looks at how his path often aligns with the traditional hero's journey, but how unusual it is that he shares much of it with his mother, Jessica. It examines him as a courageous and skilled fighter, as well as someone who possesses both masculine and feminine traits due to his genetics and training. The chapter also discusses how Paul appears as a cautious thinker and savior figure who faces numerous limitations, and that his failure to prevent the jihad he foresees points to Herbert's larger warning about the dangers of charismatic heroes.

Keywords Science fiction • Frank Herbert • Hero • Masculinity • Archetype • Jihad

On the surface, *Dune* is a heroic adventure story of an extraordinary young man who must face his destiny and claim his rightful place in the world. We watch as he encounters challenges, grows in knowledge, and matures into a leader. He is honorable and loyal, sympathetic to the plight of the oppressed, and willing to help others achieve their goals while he pursues his own. But he is also more complex than most traditional heroes. He embraces a combination of masculine and feminine traits and shares

© The Author(s), under exclusive license to Springer Nature Switzerland AG 2022
K. Kennedy, *Frank Herbert's* Dune, Palgrave Science Fiction and Fantasy: A New Canon,
https://doi.org/10.1007/978-3-031-13935-2_5

his journey with his influential mother. Rather than raising up humanity, he uses religious manipulation to position himself as a messiah which then ushers in the coming of a destructive war. He is the most capable, the most gifted, and the most powerful character, but also the one to upset the balance of the universe rather than restore it. In this chapter, we explore some of the ways Paul Atreides does and does not align with the hero archetype and stereotypical characteristics of masculinity. We look at his strengths and limitations, and how he is often not in control of his journey or his gifts in spite of his growing power. We also look at the role Paul's character plays in Herbert's critique of heroes and messianic figures.

Archetypal Hero

In many ways, Paul can be considered an archetypal hero, as described by Joseph Campbell in his book *The Hero with a Thousand Faces* (1949). Campbell believed there was a monomyth, or one universal myth, that appeared in different forms in folk tales, legends, and stories across the world. Also known as the hero's journey, the monomyth includes a set of standard features. The hero generally goes on a quest or adventure, undergoes various tests and trials, and returns with something to benefit their community. At each phase of the hero's adventure—departure, initiation, and return—there are typical incidents that occur, such as receiving the call to adventure, acquiring a boon, and recrossing the threshold. Paul's departure from Caladan, initiation into the Fremen's culture, and return to become emperor mirror this hero's journey [1, p. 563].

There are also common characteristics of the hero, including a special birth, exile or orphaning as a child, possession of special gifts, and desire to make an impact. Paul is the unexpected Kwisatz Haderach of the Bene Gesserit's long-term breeding program, is exiled from Caladan to Arrakis and partially orphaned when his father is killed, gains access to prescience, and desires to reclaim his dukedom and free the Fremen from their oppressors [2, p. 32]. We know from the beginning of the book that Paul is destined for something great. Not only do we see him withstand more pain in Reverend Mother Mohiam's test of humanness than any girl, we have Princess Irulan's opening epigraph which describes Paul in a legendary way as someone who has already been studied and written about, though under a different name: Muad'Dib. This provides a sense that he has already become a legend and that we are going back to learn about his journey.

Like most heroes throughout history and literature, Paul is male and showcases several stereotypical characteristics of masculinity from the culture he represents. When we think about the traits traditionally associated with masculinity in Western culture, for example, we might list bravery, courage, strength, honor, and toughness. Masculinity is defined in opposition to femininity, creating sets of opposite traits such as hard/soft, thinking/feeling, and rational/irrational. These stereotypes can make it difficult for authors to develop well-rounded characters who show a range of traits and emotions, since male characters who have too many traits of femininity may be seen in negative terms as effeminate or weak. Part of what makes Paul a more complex heroic character is that sometimes he is very aligned to the archetypal hero and traditional masculinity, but at other times he breaks the mold. This supports Herbert's interest in showing us as readers a more nuanced and critical view of heroes, if we are paying attention.

The most obvious way Paul fulfills an ideal of traditional masculinity is through becoming a skilled fighter and leveraging that to gain power and leadership. Paul is "*a fighting machine born and trained to it from infancy*" [3, p. 304]. Under the guidance of his weapons master, Duncan Idaho, and Gurney Halleck, he learns how to fight with weapons and shields. He also learns the 'weirding way' of the Bene Gesserit from his mother, which includes techniques for engaging in unarmed combat. These prepare him to engage in single-hand combat to the death with the Fremen man Jamis, and his victory begins his successful initiation into the tribe. Although Jessica attempts to prevent him from growing to enjoy killing by speaking harshly to him, hoping for him to associate it with something shameful, it is not long before Paul engages in regular killing as he continues on the hero's journey and steps into the shoes of a leader. On his raids with the Fremen, Paul adds guerrilla warfare to his skillset and amasses a following of death commandos, called Fedaykin, and a reputation as a fierce warrior. In many ways, Paul becomes a Lawrence of Arabia type of leader—an outsider who gains insider status and imparts his knowledge to help an oppressed people fight while maintaining his allegiance to an imperial power. His transformation moves him away from the image of an innocent young man burdened by killing a stranger, and toward a strategic leader hardened to the realities of struggling against another military power. His insistence on responding to Feyd-Rautha Harkonnen's challenge himself also creates a final showdown between the two young noblemen that highlights the physical nature of conflict in Herbert's universe (see Fig. 5.1).

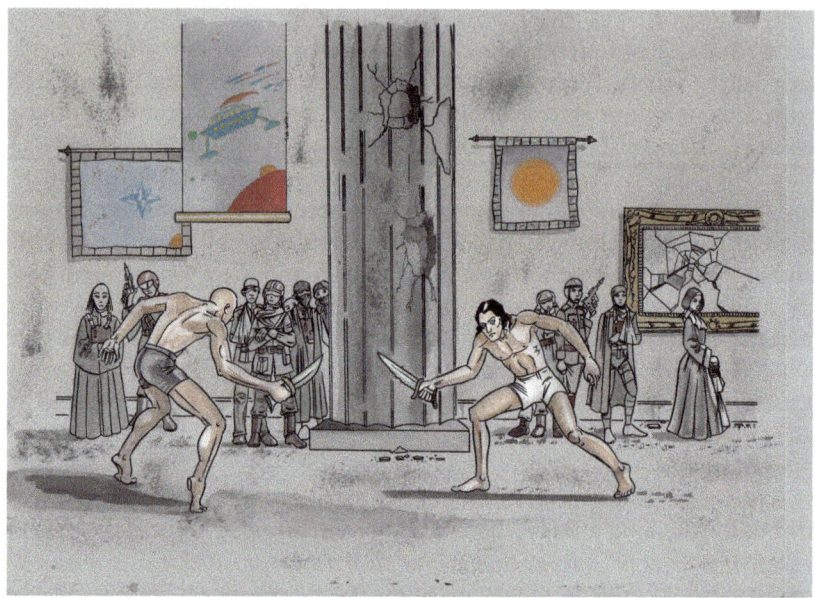

Fig. 5.1 Feyd-Rautha Harkonnen and Paul Atreides face off in a knife fight. *Reproduced with permission from illustrator Arthur Whelan*

However, there is also a notable example of the book both perpetuating and critiquing the idea of the courageous fighter, almost simultaneously. As Paul fills the vacuum left by Liet-Kynes and gains acceptance as the leader of the Fremen, this threatens the very man who has helped him reach this achievement, Stilgar. According to Fremen tradition, Paul should challenge Stilgar's leadership through single combat. But Paul makes room for an alternative view by suggesting that this tradition is flawed for weakening the Fremen in the face of their enemies. Instead of following this tradition, he dramatically puts on his father's ducal ring, which he swore to only do when he was ready to reclaim his dukedom, and asks Stilgar to kneel and pledge his loyalty to Paul as the Duke. Paul's action thus critiques the cult of masculinity that demands men fight each other to see who is the strongest, but still reinforces his male claim to be the ruler of a planet within a patriarchal hierarchy.

Paul's courage and skill in fighting are important features of his character, but his overriding characteristic is being a cautious thinker who carefully considers his actions. When we first meet him, he is lying awake in bed, his mind whirling with new knowledge as he considers the strange words he has overhead from Reverend Mother Mohiam. Throughout the rest of the story, we see him continue this behavior of analyzing things around him and wondering about his environment, his dreams, his visions, and his future. For instance, when the hunter-seeker appears in his room, his mind flashes with knowledge of its limitations before he determines how to react. When his father says Paul must decide whether to continue with Mentat training, Paul sees an omen of death in Leto's smile and feels the terrible purpose reawaken within him. As discussed in Chap. 4, the nature of Herbert's narrative style means we often have access to Paul's internal thoughts and can watch him wrestling with decisions and thinking anxiously about the future. He is a hyperconscious character, like his mother. This focuses our attention on him as a thinker, a cerebral hero who relies on the strength of his mind in addition to his body. At its heart, *Dune* is centered on the mind and the development of Paul's mental powers [4, p. 87]. The physical skills are a means to an end.

Paul is also depicted as having a consensual, monogamous relationship, which showcases his honorable nature and sets him apart from the villainous Harkonnen. Aside from their physical appearance, one of the key differences between the Baron and Paul relates to their sexuality. Paul appears to be a model young man who gains an intimate female partner in Chani and treats her with respect and love. They become life partners who care for and support one another even though they are from very different cultures. Chani acts as his confidante and advisor, in addition to bearing and raising their young son. We see Paul's strong devotion shine through when he vows that he will not allow his political marriage with another woman, Princess Irulan, to affect his relationship with Chani, though he also appears to be motivated by a desire to keep closer control of his lineage. Like his father, he remains committed to his concubine even while using marriage or the prospect of marriage for political purposes. This depiction of the hero's love for one woman demonstrates he is an honorable and trustworthy man.

In contrast, the Baron is portrayed as a pedophile who rapes young, drugged, slave boys and has no interest in women. He frequently comments on the lovely nature of boys' bodies, including Paul's and Feyd-Rautha's, which adds an element of incest into the picture. His sexual hunger appears limitless, like his physical hunger. The "crudely worked-through homophobia" and Otherness in the Baron's characterization date the book, though it can be argued it is the non-consensual nature of the Baron's sexual desires that truly make him a villain [5, p. 42]. His dislike of women was not an insurmountable problem for the Bene Gesserit and their breeding program, for they somehow managed to seduce him in order to obtain a child with his genetic material. However, aside from this instance, the Baron disavows the Bene Gesserit, which places him at a large disadvantage because he cannot benefit from their advice or training as the Atreides do. Meanwhile, Feyd-Rautha is a promiscuous young man who keeps a pleasure house full of slave women, whom he is forced to slaughter as punishment for his assassination attempt on the Baron. Neither man seems to want or be able to have sexual relationships free from slavery or coercion. Their mode of operation is to use and abuse others, sexually and otherwise, which makes Paul stand out even further as an honorable character.

Departure from the Archetype

There are several important ways in which Paul does not completely align with the hero archetype, however. For one, he receives significant support and guidance from his mother. In this way, Herbert changes the structure of the heroic journey by having a woman share in the hero's role and participate in much of the adventure along with the hero [2, p. 31; 6, p. 174]. We can see that Jessica is actively engaged in Paul's adventure at almost every step. She allows him to undergo the test of humanness and have discussions with Reverend Mother Mohiam. She helps pave the way for him to be viewed as the Fremen's savior figure. She continues training him in the Bene Gesserit Way and prana-bindu on Arrakis. And they both train the Fremen in the Bene Gesserit way of combat so they can take on the Harkonnen and then Sardaukar forces. She is not a mere background character but a full participant helping to drive the story. Her critical role must be considered when discussing Paul's journey as a heroic figure, for he is by no means a self-made young man.

Another interesting feature of Paul is that he possesses both masculine and feminine traits. Part of this is due to the combination of training he receives. On the one hand, he receives intensive training in the Bene Gesserit Way and learns how to master consciousness and abilities such as the Voice. On the other hand, he receives Mentat training that helps him process data quickly and efficiently. These trainings are not necessarily feminine or masculine in and of themselves. However, because the Bene

Gesserit are a female order and only men are shown as Mentats, the trainings can be viewed as representing different types of education that together make a more powerful whole. Paul combines Mentat calculation abilities with Bene Gesserit sensitivities to minute details, with the added layer of the spice drug, to achieve his extraordinary prescient awareness [7, p. 73].

The more important explanation for Paul's nature is the uniqueness of his genes. As the end-product of the Bene Gesserit's breeding program, Paul as the Kwisatz Haderach was intended to be a hybrid figure—a male Bene Gesserit who could see into the past and the future. In this way, he would combine the masculine and feminine elements of the psyche that were theorized by psychologist Carl Jung. Jung's influence appears clearly in the language Paul uses after coming out of his weeks-long spice-induced coma:

> There is in each of us an ancient force that takes and an ancient force that gives. A man finds little difficulty facing that place within himself where the taking force dwells, but it's almost impossible for him to see into the giving force without changing into something other than man. For a woman, the situation is reversed. [3, p. 445]

When Jessica asks him whether he is the giver or taker, he replies, "I'm at the fulcrum," signaling that he has found a psychic balance with his newfound awareness [3, p. 445]. Paul is thus positioned as a hero who merges the dualities of masculine and feminine. Rather than rejecting the feminine element, he embraces it and gains strength as a result.

But the Jungian connection becomes problematic in terms of its division of masculine and feminine capabilities. Although Jungian scholars may note that these are not absolutely limited to males and females, this is the impression given in *Dune*. Paul is special because as a male he can access both masculine and feminine sides of the psyche. Certainly, we can see that Paul appears to have more power than the Bene Gesserit since he can go into the dark space in the unconscious that repels and terrorizes them. He can look where the Bene Gesserit cannot—"into both feminine and masculine pasts" [3, p. 13]. Yet although there are gendered aspects to consider in the abilities of the hero as compared to those of other characters, these are not as straightforward as they might seem. The book is inconsistent with regard to the division of male and female in terms of psychic strength or special prescient abilities. Reverend Mother Ramallo's indication that only females are strong enough to withstand the psychic pairing in the Water of Life ceremony makes them appear to be stronger and more capable than males. Both Reverend Mother Mohiam and Alia appear to have some kind of abilities related to the future, but with no explanations given, we remain in the dark about their full extent. This adds to the mystery of the Bene Gesserit but may also make us question why they cannot or do not have the kind of prescience they hope to find through their breeding program.

LIMITATIONS OF THE HERO

Like some heroes, Paul faces limitations because he has already been set on a pre-determined path. But if we look closely, we see just how few choices he actually has. Bene Gesserit breeding, training, and missionary work have set up Paul to become not only the Kwisatz Haderach but a full messianic figure. He is primed to have his consciousness invaded by visions and have the people of Arrakis revere him as a kind of savior. Mentat training has set Paul up to handle large amounts of information and continually process and analyze it at a higher level than ordinary people. As a Mentat, he cannot help seeing the world through calculations and logical probabilities. Meanwhile, both his parents encourage him to capitalize on the Fremen's belief in order to protect himself and recruit troops. Their political savviness becomes his, almost as a matter of course. Finally, the spice unlocks more visions of the future to the point that he lives life according to his time-vision and has trouble distinguishing dream from reality. His frustration with imperfect prescience drives him to the dangerous decision to take the Water of Life like his mother, thus fulfilling his destiny to become a male Bene Gesserit. His prescience turns him into a superhuman, but it becomes a curse from which he cannot escape [8, p. 70]. Thus, Paul is not often in control of his journey or his gifts. All of his hard work in training his mind and body and striving to live up to his parents' hopes for him serve to further lock him into a journey that he foresees will end in an uncontrollable jihad.

A complex topic about doctrines and practices relating to both internal and external struggles across the span of Islamic history, jihad has become a more loaded term since the time of *Dune*'s publication. In the book, the term is used to refer to both the crusade against computers in the distant past and a religious war yet to come, and Paul's inability to prevent the latter demonstrates a severe limitation of his character as a hero and a messiah. Throughout his journey we see Paul wrestle with the knowledge that one of the paths he could take leads to a jihad that sweeps across the universe. In the stilltent with his mother, he sees two main branchings: one leading to him confronting Baron Harkonnen and the other leading to a warrior religion spreading across the universe. He labels the latter a jihad, the ancient way of renewing humanity's bloodlines, but thinks, "*Surely, I cannot choose that way*" [3, p. 199]. After killing Jamis, he again has a vision of a future with "the jihad's bloody swords and fanatic legions" [3, p. 309]. He even blames the Fremen for trying to ensnare him in "the wild jihad, the religious war he felt he should avoid at any cost" [3, p. 347]. Yet "[t]he more he resisted his terrible purpose and fought against the coming of the jihad, the greater the turmoil that wove through his prescience" [3, p. 388].

The jihad is presented as an inevitable result of Paul taking up the mantle of the messiah of the Fremen and deliberately using religion as a tool to unify his forces. Just as Liet-Kynes secures the Fremen's loyalty through convincing them to believe in a dream of Dune as a paradise, Paul gains their loyalty through styling himself as the most skilled fighter and their long-awaited messiah. While both characters rely on the power of a shared vision, Paul benefits from drumming up religious fervor to ensure he has access to a cohesive fighting force. His use of religion and the allusion to a looming jihad, in particular, link the circumstances in *Dune* with historic events when the concept of a jihad or holy war was used to unite people toward a shared goal. For instance, in the early years of Islam, the emerging doctrine of jihad was used as a way of maintaining unity among Arab tribes, and in the fight against Russian imperialists in the 1800s, holy war was used by the Islamic brotherhood known as the Murīdīs to unite dissenting mountain tribes [9, p. 28; 10]. In November 1914, after the start of World War I, Ottoman Sultan-Caliph Mehmed v Reshad proclaimed a jihad, calling upon the Muslim subjects of Russia, Britain, and France to resist their oppressors and not join in the war against the Ottoman state [11, p. 14].

Part of Herbert's critique of religion, the jihad then represents the danger when politics and religion combine to become an unstoppable, disruptive force. Through Paul and the Fremen, Herbert highlights the incredible ability of religion to shape human beliefs and behaviors, while also showing its destructive side and the difficulty in keeping it under control. Despite arrogantly believing he alone can prevent this catastrophe, Paul finds himself swept along in the path of consequences triggered by other people's decisions and desires. Unlike other heroes who are convinced they are right, Paul is a reluctant hero who in the end realizes he is fallible and unable to control the outcomes of his actions as a leader [8, p. 73]. It is only before his fight with Feyd-Rautha at the end of the book that Paul accepts that his efforts were futile, and that he was the one to show the Fremen the way and give them the mastery over the Guild they would need to leave Arrakis and unleash the jihad.

It is a tragic irony that Paul is so powerful yet helpless in the face of the jihad. This is one signal that the hero's journey in *Dune* is more of a tragedy than a success story. The parallels with Greek tragedy further confirm this reading. Paul belongs to House Atreides, whose name alludes to the Greek myth of the House of Atreus, which was cursed with intergenerational dynastic violence [1, p. 561]. There are several family killings in *Dune*: the Baron kills Leto (partner to his granddaughter), Alia kills the Baron (her grandfather), and Paul kills Feyd-Rautha (his cousin). Furthermore, Leto's name links him with the goddess Leto, mother of Apollo and Artemis. Thus, we may view Paul as an Apollo figure who gains abilities in prophecy and combat, but can also bring plague upon his enemies, as Apollo does in the *Iliad* [1, pp. 570–571]. In Paul's case, though, he brings about a type of plague upon the whole universe. His grasping of psychological and political power solves nothing for humanity, which is denied the ability to control its own destiny [12, p. 11]. The parallels between the stories in *Dune* and Greek drama, particular Aeschylus' tragedy, *Oresteia*, suggest that Paul does not bring a boon back to his community at the end of his journey, but a curse in the form of the jihad [1, p. 571].

CRITICISM OF HEROES

Whether or not readers pick up on Paul's anxiety about the jihad or the allusions to Greek myths, they can find other subtle critiques of heroes and messianic figures throughout *Dune*. Paul's shift from a naïve young nobleman into a battle-hardened guerrilla fighter demonstrates the corruptive effect of seeking power. When Duke Leto tries to explain to Paul how he wins loyalty as a leader through cultivating an air of bravura and having a robust propaganda program, Paul protests at his father's cynical attitude to governing. Paul wants to believe men follow his father willingly out of love. It appears Paul has not accepted his despondent father's belief, that "Power and fear" are the "tools of statecraft" [3, p. 105]. However, over the course of the novel, we see this idealistic young man gradually come to accept his father's advice about training in guerrilla fighting. His raids with the Fremen help build him up to be a legendary leader who supposedly orders battle drums to be made from the skins of his enemies. Paul's shift to becoming an inspirational guerrilla warrior signals his development into a leader who accepts the view that to rule means to seize power and instill fear when necessary. As discussed in Chap. 4, Paul also gradually loses touch with his emotions and discards his father's value of human life.

Paul's insistence on cultivating a religious bravura to take hold of and maintain power presents a cautionary message about the role of messianic figures. Paul follows both of his parents' advice in capitalizing on the people's belief that he is their Mahdi, their Lisan al-Gaib. He relies on his prescient visions and special training to help deliberately style himself as their long-awaited messiah. Yet eventually even Jessica becomes fearful of Paul's indoctrination of the Fremen to unite the forces under himself as a religious leader and cautions him of the danger in this path. Coming from the perspective of not only his mother, but a Bene Gesserit who is very aware of the power of religious indoctrination, this warning should hold significant weight. However, Paul brushes aside her concern by noting that she taught him this way of operating. It is what he sees as the pathway to leadership on Arrakis and he will not be dissuaded. Close to his final victory over his enemies, Paul realizes "how Stilgar had been transformed from the Fremen naib to a *creature* of the Lisan al-Gaib, a receptacle for awe and obedience. It was a lessening of the man" [3, p. 469]. A significant consequence of Paul's religious indoctrination has been that the Fremen have become worshippers rather than friends, beholden to the messianic myth rather than seeing and reasoning clearly. He has lessened their status as individuals and as a people in the name of his quest to reclaim power.

There is also a warning message in the ecologist Liet-Kynes seeming to regret his part in enabling Paul to become a hero figure among the Fremen. As a John the Baptist figure, Liet-Kynes plays a key role in paving the way for Paul's acceptance among the Fremen. He carefully evaluates Paul and is swayed by his personality and pledge of loyalty, as well as various signs that Paul is the one foretold in the messianic legends. Yet as he is left for dead in the desert after helping Paul and Jessica escape the Harkonnen, Kynes hallucinates his father saying: "No more terrible disaster could befall your people than for them to fall into the hands of a Hero" [3, p. 276]. Liet-Kynes then reflects on how he has already put out a command for the Fremen to find and protect Paul, and this may have set in motion a completely different potential than the one he and his father had been working toward. His dying thoughts offer a poignant warning to the reader that there is danger brewing with Paul, though he is but a boy. "Appendix I: The Ecology of Dune", too, ends on an ominous note: "The course had been set by this time, the Ecological-Fremen were aimed along their way. Liet-Kynes had only to watch and nudge and spy upon the Harkonnens ... until the day his planet was afflicted by a Hero" [3, p. 500]. The explicit use of the term Hero (with a capital H) shows that Herbert as an author is fully aware of Paul being set up as the hero archetype and at the same time is critical of this concept. The words "terrible disaster" and "afflicted" clearly indicate some kind of threat to the usual order. Here, Paul is treated like a thing that will negatively impact the Fremen and the ecological project, rather than a person who will heroically save them.

Complex Heroes

The archetypal hero figure in *Dune* is not what he at first seems, and the multi-faceted nature of his character helped pave the way for more complex heroes in science fiction. In Paul, Herbert offers a twist on the hero we expect to find. He is bred and trained to be a duke's heir, but also a male Bene Gesserit with special prescient powers. He embodies traditional characteristics of masculinity such as being courageous and a strong fighter, but also embraces the Bene Gesserit Way and the feminine side of the psyche. He has various male tutors and companions, yet takes the hero's journey with his mother at his side. Importantly, though, despite all of his special abilities, he is a hero who is not in full control of them and ultimately fails to prevent the destructive jihad he foresees. Paul shows that the good guy can get it wrong [8, p. 71]. Emerging in the postwar period of the U.S., he reflects a shattering of hope in righteous and ideal heroes who save the innocent [8, p. 73]. Complex heroes would become more prominent in science fiction as well as fantasy in the following decades. Authors placed more uncertainty and ambivalence in their heroes, showed behavior that was not always heroic, and demonstrated the sometimes negative consequences of their intervention in the world [8, p. 79]. This increase in sophistication has enabled heroes to continue to appeal to modern audiences, and the hunger for these kinds of characters shows no sign of diminishing.

Another significant feature of *Dune* is the emphasis on Paul spending so much time thinking and processing as opposed to using physical abilities or technologies. This reflects part of the shift toward 'soft' science fiction happening in the genre during the mid-twentieth century, as discussed in Chap. 4. Herbert expanded on the concept of the cerebral superhero that authors such as A.E. Van Vogt were writing about and proved that mental and psychic strength could be just as interesting as physical strength [13, pp. 171–172]. Herbert also innovated on the origins of these strengths, making characters work for their superhuman abilities rather than be given them [8, p. 67].

Dune's critique of heroes and messianic leaders remains relevant today. Communication channels may change, manipulation tactics may become murkier, but people seeking power continue to appear. The fact that we may miss the warning signs, as many do with Paul, indicates how easy it is to fall for the charisma of these figures. If we look at the Fremen, we may see some of ourselves—wanting someone to make life easier for us but unaware of the high price we will pay. *Dune* suggests there are no easy answers to the problem of charismatic leaders and heroes. They will spring up in fertile soil and try to manipulate and control those around them. Even if their intentions are noble, they will become corrupt as they gain more power.

Though Paul is by no means a feminine figure, his incorporation of feminine elements through his Bene Gesserit training and his genes points to the positive potential of a less restrictive view of masculinity. Notions of masculinity in Western societies have undergone some shifts since the mid-twentieth century, but many restrictive norms continue to exist. In *Dune*, Paul is able to become more powerful than other highly skilled characters because he has been birthed by a Bene Gesserit woman as part of a special breeding program, trained by her in mind–body control and skills such as the Voice, and guided by her as he matures from boy to man. His rejection of the Bene Gesserit's control is not a rejection of women, nor of their training—he does not appear to be threatened by his Bene Gesserit influence. His characterization thus opens rather than closes the possibility that a broader view of masculinity is preferable.

References

1. Rogers, Brett M. "'Now Harkonnen Shall Kill Harkonnen': Aeschylus, Dynastic Violence, and Twofold Tragedies in Frank Herbert's *Dune*." *Brill's Companion to the Reception of Aeschylus*, edited by Rebecca Futo Kennedy, Brill, 2018, pp. 553–581.
2. Palumbo, Donald E. *A Dune Companion: Characters, Places and Terms in Frank Herbert's Original Six Novels*. McFarland, 2018.
3. Herbert, Frank. *Dune*. 1965. Berkley, 1984.
4. Manlove, C.N. "Frank Herbert, *Dune* (1965)." *Science Fiction: Ten Explorations*. Macmillan Press, 1986, pp. 79–99.
5. Roberts, Adam. "Case Study: Frank Herbert, *Dune* (1965)." *Science Fiction*. Routledge, 2000, pp. 36–46.
6. Hourihan, Margery. *Deconstructing the Hero: Literary Theory and Children's Literature*. Routledge, 1997.
7. O'Reilly, Timothy. *Frank Herbert*. Frederick Ungar, 1981.
8. Prieto-Pablos, Juan A. "The Ambivalent Hero of Contemporary Fantasy and Science Fiction." *Extrapolation*, vol. 32, no. 1, 1991, pp. 64–80.
9. Armstrong, Karen. *Holy War: The Crusades and Their Impact on Today's World*. Macmillan, 1988.
10. Blanch, Lesley. *The Sabres of Paradise: Conquest and Vengeance in the Caucasus*. John Murray, 1960.
11. Zürcher, Erik-Jan. "Introduction: The Ottoman Jihad, the German Jihad and the Sacralization of War." *Jihad and Islam in World War I: Studies on the Ottoman Jihad on the Centenary of Snouck Hurgronje's "Holy War Made in Germany,"* edited by Erik-Jan Zürcher, Leiden University Press, 2016, pp. 13–27.
12. Klein, Gérard, D. Suvin, and Leila Lecorps. "Discontent in American Science Fiction." *Science Fiction Studies*, vol. 4, no. 1, 1977, pp. 3–13.
13. Ashley, Mike. *Transformations: The Story of the Science Fiction Magazines from 1950 to 1970*. Liverpool University Press, 2005.

CHAPTER 6

Women's Influence and Control

Abstract This chapter examines the depiction of women in *Dune* and the amount of agency or control they have. It focuses on three key avenues of agency—religious, embodied, and political—as the most prominently featured for female characters operating in a feudal, male-dominated universe. The chapter looks at how the Bene Gesserit Sisterhood is modeled after the Catholic Church and uses religion as a tool, and how the Fremen grant religious authority to women. It discusses Bene Gesserit women's high level of bodily control, seen through their many abilities like the Voice, and their avenues of political control as they seek to shape the future. It also discusses the role of Jessica as a strong mother figure alongside Paul.

Keywords Science fiction • Frank Herbert • Women • Feminism • Religion • Female body

The men in *Dune* have power and control, but so do the women. Theirs is just often through different channels. Women rely on ways they have often used to be influential in male-dominated cultures. They use religion as a means of claiming wisdom and authority. They embrace their role in child-bearing and mothering. They insert themselves into the levels of

© The Author(s), under exclusive license to Springer Nature Switzerland AG 2022
K. Kennedy, *Frank Herbert's* Dune, Palgrave Science Fiction and Fantasy: A New Canon,
https://doi.org/10.1007/978-3-031-13935-2_6

official hierarchies so they are well-positioned to dispense advice and make changes favorable to themselves and other women. Everything is a potential political opportunity to be leveraged toward their ultimate goals. Although the women of *Dune* may be situated in traditional roles as mothers, partners, and advisors, they are playing the long game. In this chapter, we explore features of women's agency, defined as their ability to choose what they do, accomplish tasks, and actively influence the outcomes of events. Agency is about having control. We look at three key avenues of agency for women: religious, embodied, and political. We also examine the complexity of the representation of women and see how the use of traditional roles does not have to limit the depiction of women as capable and authoritative figures.

Religious Agency

An important aspect of female authority and power in *Dune* revolves around religion. While men have dominated mainstream religions throughout recorded history, there have been successful attempts by women to gain some measure of status through religion. For instance, women in Catholicism historically led communities of religious followers and presided over convents, though the Church increasingly restricted women's movements and pressed for more oversight by male leaders. Even while men have justified their religious superiority by pointing to male personifications of deities, male prophets, and male-dominated holy texts, women have continued to clamor for positions of religious authority that acknowledge their right to participate meaningfully in religion, with or without male approval.

Thus, it seems logical that Herbert models the Bene Gesserit Sisterhood in a religious fashion, considering that women gathering together so deliberately for other reasons might not fit within his feudal universe of emperors and male-controlled guilds. Herbert also infuses his book with the Islamic-based religious beliefs of the Fremen, discussed in Chap. 2, and places women at the top of this religious hierarchy. In fact, virtually no man asserts any religious claim to authority until the Fremen recognize Paul as their messiah, and then he is only able to lead because the Bene Gesserit planted a messianic myth among the Fremen centuries earlier. Excluding Paul's special case, then, religion is the dominion of women. The Bene Gesserit use it to hide their imperialist political project, Jessica self-consciously performs its customs to secure safety in a foreign land, and

Chani ritualistically follows it to carry on her tribe's communal traditions. Herbert gives these female characters religion as a means to assert authority in a socially acceptable manner, giving them an avenue to assume agency and power in a feudal society.

The entire set-up of the Sisterhood is a twist on what women could traditionally achieve in a feudal society. Herbert provides women with their own organization which is free to operate as it wishes and pursue political projects without male oversight. Rather than openly announce their aspirations for power, the Bene Gesserit cloak themselves in religion as a convenient method of secrecy. It remains doubtful whether or not the Sisterhood even constitutes a religious organization, for outsiders and we as readers learn little of what beliefs and teachings actually exist at its schools. "Appendix II: The Religion of Dune" describes the sisters as members "who privately denied they were a religious order, but who operated behind an almost impenetrable screen of ritual mysticism, and whose training, whose symbolism, organization, and internal teaching methods were almost wholly religious" [1, pp. 500–501]. The Bene Gesserit seem to have latched onto religious mysticism because it enables them to appear non-threatening to outsiders and efficiently train women. According to the small pieces of information given on their schools, they compare with Catholic convents where women are set apart from men, donning dark habits and learning to submit themselves to their studies [2, p. 15]. Unlike convents, though, the schools and indeed the whole organization are completely populated and managed by women. No male overseers make restrictions or hand down orders; the Bene Gesserit dictate their own agenda to their members.

What constitutes the Sisterhood's mission is not the worship of a deity but the creation of their own god-like figure. The Bene Gesserit are devoted to conducting their breeding program and an ambiguous goal of improving humankind. Their motto—"I am Bene Gesserit: I exist only to serve"—correctly describes the loyalty demanded of members, but it obscures the fact that members are essentially serving a secret political cause rather than a religious movement [1, p. 23]. They hope to produce a male Bene Gesserit, or Kwisatz Haderach, who can gain access to both feminine and masculine memories and bridge space and time through prescient visions. It can be inferred that the Sisterhood plans to train this man to become as loyal as any female member and leverage his abilities for their own ends. They clearly grant themselves a great deal of authority by aspiring to better humanity through their genetic maneuvers; they aim to act like a god rather than worship one. The Bene Gesserit bide their time for centuries under the guise of religion, all the while covertly preparing for the day when they can assert more overt power through their genetic superhuman.

Through their missionary work, the Bene Gesserit enable members such as Jessica to use religion as a tool to secure safety and gain authority. We see her easily slip into an authoritative religious position granted by the Missionaria Protectiva's work when she faces her first dangerous encounter with the Fremen housekeeper, the Shadout Mapes, on Dune. After encountering Stilgar's tribe, she inspires the Fremen to chant along with her. She clearly knows the sayings and patterns of the Missionaria Protectiva well enough to adapt them to any situation and is well-aware of her manipulation [2, p. 155]. When Stilgar honors her with the title given to holy women, Sayyadina, she muses, "*If only he knew the tricks we use! She must've been good, that Bene Gesserit of the Missionaria Protectiva. These Fremen are beautifully prepared to believe in us*" [1, p. 284].

What solidifies Jessica and Paul's acceptance into the Fremen tribe is her undertaking of the dangerous Water of Life ceremony which proves that she is capable of taking on the highest religious position as a Reverend Mother. In spite of their religion's similarity with Islam, which in most cases denies women positions of leadership, the Fremen wholeheartedly accept women as strong, capable religious leaders. It is therefore testament to Jessica's strong religious performance that, as an outsider, she is allowed the chance to become such an integral member of the Fremen's religion. Like an abbess of a convent, Jessica utilizes her position to gain authority and respect in her new domain. She is consulted as an advisor in major decisions and maintains a network of Sayyadina spies to provide her with information. But perhaps the greatest example of her religious power comes when she prevents the Fremen, including Paul's loyal Fedaykin death commandos, from pronouncing her son dead and taking his water in the death ritual after he goes into a coma upon secretly ingesting the poisonous Water of Life.

Chani also showcases the religious authority granted to women among the Fremen. Before Jessica undergoes the ritual, Chani is consecrated as a Sayyadina in the event that Jessica fails. This situation helps clarify the difference in religious positions: the Sayyadina are religious women who hold authority and preside over certain tribal rituals but have not taken the Water of Life. Thus, Sayyadina Chani guides Jessica through the dangerous ceremony and retains a religious position herself even after Jessica succeeds. Stilgar demonstrates his awe for the religious Fremen women when he tells Jessica, "'the Sayyadina, when they are not the formal leaders, hold a special place of honor. They teach. They maintain the strength of God here.' He touched his breast" [1, p. 293]. Chani also presides over another ritual, that of Paul's worm-riding test, indicating that women maintain a role in important affairs even if they are not themselves participating in them. Chani's religious authority gives her character more dimension than if she had solely been Paul's concubine. Both Chani and Jessica serve as examples of women in *Dune* finding authority through a religious avenue.

Embodied Agency

Embodied agency is another significant feature of the representation of women in *Dune*. The women of the Bene Gesserit actually have a level of bodily control unparalleled by any man. Inwardly, they can control things such as pregnancy and can neutralize poisons in their body. Outwardly, they can use the Voice to control people and use combat skills to take out their enemies. Fremen women, too, have fierce fighting skills, which are enhanced once they receive additional combat training from Jessica and Paul. Although many characters in the book seem to be largely unaware of women's skills, we as readers can piece together the full picture of the embodied agency that Herbert gives them.

Historically, women were largely responsible for issues regarding pregnancy and birth, enlisting the help of midwives for advice and labor assistance. But with the introduction of the male-dominated medical establishment and the increasing use of medical technology, many women found their knowledge and experience dismissed. Writing in the 1960s, when reproductive technology was still in its infancy, Herbert envisions a universe where women are in complete control. But the Bene Gesserit's control over reproduction is so understated that many readers overlook it and its significance. It is only through subtle hints that we can speculate that Bene Gesserit women can choose both when to become pregnant and what sex of child to conceive [2, p. 76]. This is first implied when Reverend Mother Mohiam considers Jessica's disobedience: "*If only she'd borne us a girl as she was ordered to do!*" [1, p. 6]. Later, during her second pregnancy, Jessica thinks to herself that her unborn daughter was "*conceived out of instinct and not out of obedience*" [1, p. 190]. This shows that even though neither of her children is born according to the Sisterhood's orders, she had the ability to exert control over her pregnancies. The ability is further implied when Princess Irulan discloses that her mother only bore daughters to the Emperor due to orders from her Sister Superiors, and when Lady Margot Fenring plans to become pregnant via Feyd-Rautha Harkonnen to secure his bloodline for the Sisterhood. The Bene Gesserit enable women to take responsibility for their own bodies, including reproductive capabilities, with no outside interference.

One critical perspective on the Bene Gesserit is that they are overly focused on reproduction and reinforce a degrading view of women as 'breeders' only useful for producing offspring. Certainly, reproductive control is portrayed as an essential part of their overall plan for humanity, and they embrace women's ability to create new life. Bene Gesserit women are subject to the demands of the Sisterhood, and their choices are largely shaped by the necessities of the genetic breeding program. For them, the good of the group outweighs individual desires. This tension would be mirrored in the real-life women's movement, as women formed collectives and faced the notion of sacrificing their personal preferences to make political statements and advance the cause of women's rights [2, p. 82]. However, women are not shown as being resentful of their participation in the long-term Bene Gesserit plan. They seem to have a solid sense of solidarity and loyalty to the organization. Furthermore, women still decide when to conceive and, ultimately, like Jessica, can disobey orders and choose whichever sex of child they want. The Bene Gesserit could be criticized if they only saw women's worth in reproduction regulated by men's technology and men's desires. But they are shown using reproductive power to control lineage and further their own larger agenda for humanity, often without men even being aware of it. Women are also shown using abilities in several areas unrelated to reproduction, as discussed below.

The Bene Gesserit's skills in using the Voice and engaging in unarmed combat are more pronounced aspects of their embodied agency. These reverse the stereotype linking men with strength and command, and women with weakness and submission (see Fig. 6.1). Through the Voice, women can control others with nothing more than their speech. For example, as mentioned in Chap. 4, when Thufir Hawat, one of Duke Leto's closest advisors, accuses Jessica of being the traitor in the Atreides' household, she uses the Voice to shock him and show how much latent power she has. Hawat's thoughts reveal his awe at her skill: "To do what she had done spoke of […] a depth of control he had not dreamed possible" [1, p. 156]. The Voice removes the element of choice from those

6 WOMEN'S INFLUENCE AND CONTROL   83

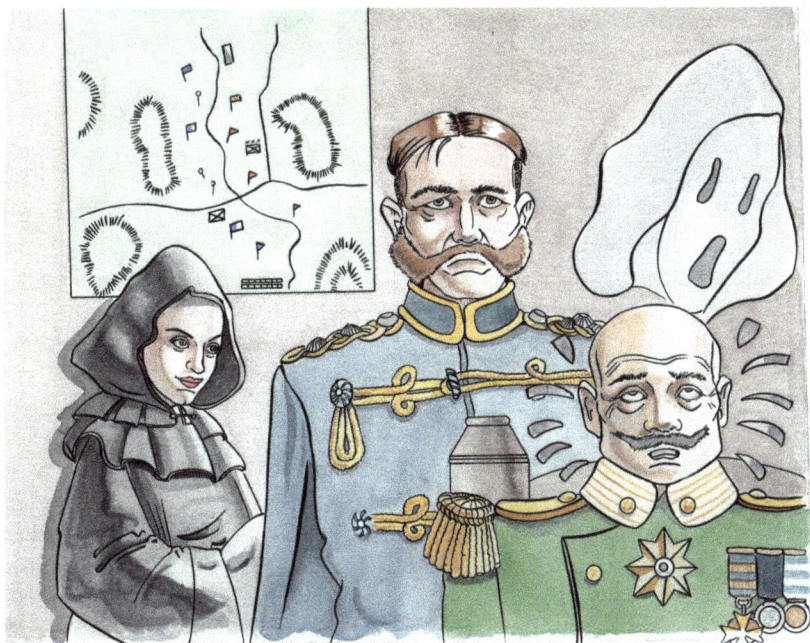

Fig. 6.1 A Bene Gesserit woman using the Voice. *Reproduced with permission from illustrator Arthur Whelan*

commanded. All human agency in this encounter is placed with the one using the Voice. Jessica voluntarily divulges the technique of the Voice to Paul; otherwise, only Bene Gesserit women hold the power to command people in such a way.

If there is no alternative but to fight for survival, the Bene Gesserit are also fully trained in hand-to-hand combat, what the Fremen call the weirding ability of battle. The extent of Jessica's combat prowess becomes clear in her encounter with the Fremen [2, p. 52]. After she realizes the military party intends to kill her and Paul for their water, her "muscles overrode all fatigue, flowed into maximum readiness without external betrayal" [1, p. 270]. Her faultless preparation in the face of danger is contrasted with Paul's hesitance; he is "less conditioned to emergency response than his mother" and must force himself to fall into "the arrested whipsnap of muscles that can slash in any direction" [1, p. 270]. Stilgar is caught off-guard by her skills: "a slash of her arm, a whirling of mingled robes, and she was against the rocks with the man helpless in front of her" [1, p. 281]. Besting the strongest man in the tribe even while unarmed convinces the Fremen of Jessica's value, and Stilgar openly states his admiration at her superior fighting ability and that he covets it for his people. For a woman's fighting skills to be so admired by the fierce warrior culture of the Fremen speaks volumes.

The Fremen offer another example of women exerting agency through combat. Fremen women and children have reputations off-world as being violent and dangerous like their men. We see young Chani traveling with Stilgar's military party, aiming a projectile weapon at Paul and clearly prepared for violence. Her initial disdain later gives way to affection, but in this first encounter Herbert shows that Fremen women are indeed strong and fierce from childhood. Even after Chani becomes Paul's concubine and respects his authority in certain matters, she still acts according to her own will. Over Paul's protests, Chani defends her decision to slay one of his challengers without consulting him. She considers herself a capable fighter and one who knows what is best for Paul, despite his prideful belief that only he should combat his challengers. Paul's young sister, Alia, also behaves in the fierce Fremen way. She assumes leadership of an attack group of Fremen women, children, and old men that almost overwhelms the Emperor's Sardaukar forces. Alia thus asserts an extraordinary level of combat agency for both a female and a child, and she shows no fear when in the captivity of the Emperor and Baron Harkonnen. In fact, she proceeds to kill the Baron with a gom jabbar, taking this act of revenge for herself and precluding Paul from it. Though the Fremen still consist of a society with male sietch leaders, their culture has adapted to desert conditions and oppression by cultivating battle-readiness among all members, whether man, woman, or child.

POLITICAL AGENCY

Although the political system in *Dune* is depicted as feudal, with men holding the official positions of power as emperors, barons, and dukes, women are still shown playing politics behind the scenes, which they have done in many civilizations. Women have historically made use of the resources at their disposal to become valuable to those in seats of power. They have often had to assert authority in covert ways to avoid being considered a threat to the patriarchal establishment. They have also played significant roles in organizing political movements and revolutions, despite being overlooked by historians. Even though they have rarely ruled in their own right and continue to lack leadership parity with men, this does not mean women lack political motivation, influence, and power. In *Dune*, the Bene Gesserit are the ones who most illustrate this concept. Appearing to believe that power is a corruptive force best handled at a distance, they find alternative avenues of political control as they seek to maneuver people and shape the future. Jessica also grasps a significant amount of political control when she acts like a regent for her son.

Herbert suggests that the Sisterhood is one of the major players in the *Dune* universe, but he does not explain how it came to acquire such status, especially being the only female group. He does, however, give some indications of how members use their status to gain political influence. The Bene Gesserit intentionally make women available as partners to high-ranking officials in order to infiltrate the households of powerful figures [2, p. 154]. Presumably, part of their strategy is to present women as well-educated and useful for noble families. Jessica herself wonders whether her business training might have played a role in Duke Leto's interest in her. Bene Gesserit women present a contrast with Mentats, who also appear to serve at the pleasure of noble households but lack the type of intimate relationship that allows for different forms of persuasion and influence. The Bene Gesserit also take advantage of the tradition of arranged marriages to secure bloodlines and the line of succession while maintaining secrecy around their ability to control reproduction. Duke Leto does not realize that Jessica is selected for him because of his Atreides genes, nor does he know that she is only supposed to bear daughters as part of a long-term breeding program. He is one of presumably many heads of noble families whose Bene Gesserit partners have certain reproductive orders. It is implied that the Bene Gesserit's goal is to produce a superhuman not merely for the improvement of the human race, but for the potential to place him on the imperial throne. Their endgame is politically motivated. What hints at the Bene Gesserit's desired political result is their severe restriction on the Emperor's progeny. The Sisterhood essentially traps the Emperor by instructing his late Bene Gesserit wife, Anirul, to bear only daughters. Their refusal to grant him a male heir aligns with their design to place their future Kwisatz Haderach on the throne [3, p. 315]. Ultimately, the Bene Gesserit's breeding program is a deeply political project.

Furthermore, by the time of *Dune*'s events, the Bene Gesserit have become invaluable by providing the Emperor with his own personal

Truthsayer, a Bene Gesserit who can detect whether people believe what they are saying or not. Reverend Mother Mohiam is feared by anyone seeking to deceive the Emperor. This justifies a major plot point in which Jessica and Paul are able to escape because the Baron does not order them to be outright killed [2, p. 122]. He *"fears the questioning of a Truthsayer"* and wants "no blood" on his hands [1, p. 165]. During the tense confrontation at the end of the book involving the Baron and Atreides family, it also becomes clear that Reverend Mother Mohiam is not merely a lie-detecting instrument, but actually the Emperor's key advisor. She takes up a position behind his throne, resting her hand on it in a signal that she holds the real power as she looms over him. When Paul's attacking forces invade the room, the Emperor retreats to a sealed chamber and turns to Reverend Mother Mohiam in desperation. It is she who issues the command to bring forth their weapon of last resort, Count Hasimir Fenring. She is also the one to persuade the Emperor to allow his daughter, Princess Irulan, to marry Paul, and remind him of the Bene Gesserit agreement with him to place one of their members on the throne. Thus, while the Emperor holds the official position of power and the authority to accede to Paul's demands, Reverend Mother Mohiam holds a notable amount of political power and influence herself.

As a Bene Gesserit, Jessica is understandably portrayed as a politically savvy woman as well. So it follows that when she and Paul are forced into exile after the Harkonnen attack, she takes up a position akin to a regent, someone who will advise and guide Paul toward reclaiming his dukedom one day. As the concubine of Duke Leto, she might be viewed as only receiving status based on her association with a high-ranking male. However, the Duke dies a third of the way into the book. Jessica takes the opportunity to secure a foothold among the Fremen as a good regent would secure a partnership with an influential ally for future stability. She initiates a pact with Stilgar to teach his tribe the weirding way of battle in exchange for safe haven. She advises Paul to accept Jamis' water after his death so that the tribe will not be offended. Then she undertakes the dangerous ceremony to become a Reverend Mother. Since the Fremen view their loyalty to Jessica and Paul not as submission but as obedience to their religious prophecy, this enables Jessica to safely pave the way for Paul to gain both religious and political legitimacy because he must arrive as the offspring of a Bene Gesserit to truly be the Fremen's long-awaited savior. Every step of the way, Jessica displays her skills in political strategy and diplomacy.

The Hero's Debt

The various religious, embodied, and political agencies asserted by women can be viewed as part of a subversive theme complementing Herbert's critique of the masculine hero ideal, discussed in Chap. 5. Rather than position Paul as a self-made man, Herbert shows how his image and skill-set have been constructed through an all-female organization's genetic control, training regime, and missionary project. It is through becoming a male Bene Gesserit that Paul secures the prescience and authority needed to succeed in the hero's journey. Herbert also places a strong mother figure at Paul's side, reminding us that women's guidance is a significant part of his development and growth. Even once Paul has emerged as the Kwisatz Haderach, poised to take the path of religious and political dominance of Dune and the Imperium, Jessica continues to act as the wise advisor who feels free to rebuke her disciple when he attempts a haughty air of superiority over her: "'I see the signs!' Jessica snapped. 'My question was meant to remind you that you should not try to teach me in those matters in which I instructed you'" [1, p. 479]. Notably, Herbert refrains from ending his epic adventure story with a grand speech or coronation of Paul as the new emperor. Rather, he shows Paul intently conversing with Jessica and Chani, asking them to negotiate with the Emperor for him and assuring them that their desires will be met. It is Jessica's speech which concludes *Dune*, with her declaration that she and Chani will be so revered as concubines that history will honor them as wives without them needing such formal status. Truly this ending points to the fact that the women of *Dune* have an influential role in the story and multiple forms of agency.

Feminist Speculation

The representation of women in *Dune* was part of a shift in science fiction toward more three-dimensional characterization for female characters as well as male ones. Unlike Robert Heinlein's *Stranger in a Strange Land* (1961)—another bestseller of the 1960s which features a male messianic figure—*Dune* devoted substantial textual space and authority to its women. It demonstrated that women did not necessarily need to be shown in radically altered roles for an author to give them complex characterization and multiple pathways to agency and control over their lives. Whereas other science fiction outsourced reproduction to male scientists or technological gadgetry or avoided it as a topic altogether, *Dune* kept it as an important part of women's experience. It also showed that a science fiction story could be successful with a leading mother figure at the side of the hero. In speculating about the future for women, it offered a seemingly simple concept: what if women were in control of their bodies and used religious and political influence to their advantage while still operating in a male-dominated society. In this way, *Dune* is a book that deals with feminist themes and helped shape the genre ahead of the flourishing of feminist science fiction in the 1970s when the second-wave women's movement reached its height.

In spite of social and cultural upheavals that have opened new doors for many women, gender norms, power dynamics, and societal expectations continue to play a large part in constraining women's bodies and lives. The expressions of women's agency in *Dune* are sometimes subtle, but perhaps they offer us a more realistic view of future progress than other science fiction stories. The likelihood is that changes in women's roles, levels of control, and influence in the real world will take place in small increments, through traditional pathways, rather than suddenly being overturned. There are more women taking up senior political positions, but they remain a small minority. There have been advances in reproductive technology, but for the foreseeable future many women will continue to bear children. There have been only limited reforms in some religions enabling women to access previously off-limits roles. *Dune* prompts us to consider how to recognize women's influence, leadership, and authority within the constraints of an unequal society.

References

1. Herbert, Frank. *Dune*. 1965. Berkley, 1984.
2. Kennedy, Kara. *Women's Agency in the* Dune *Universe: Tracing Women's Liberation through Science Fiction*. Palgrave Macmillan, 2021.
3. DiTommaso, Lorenzo. "History and Historical Effect in Frank Herbert's 'Dune.'" *Science Fiction Studies*, vol. 19, no. 3, 1992, pp. 311–325.

CHAPTER 7

A Complex World

Abstract This concluding chapter provides an overview of other interesting avenues of interpretation of *Dune*, some of which have not yet been well-explored in the scholarship. Perspectives that have received some attention include those from philosophy, classical studies, and comparative literature, while emerging areas of study include world-building, linguistics, translation studies, postcolonialism, and posthumanism. The chapter concludes by discussing *Dune*'s ambiguity and openness to multiple interpretations, which make it ripe for new critical perspectives and debates.

Keywords Science fiction • Dune • Frank Herbert • World-building

Dune is undoubtedly a complex book. Published in the 1960s, it has proved its continuing relevance with classic themes and considerable depth underlying the main storyline of a young hero seeking to reclaim his title. This study has examined several key features and approaches that elevate it to a literary masterpiece, but there are many more. This final chapter touches on other interesting avenues of interpretation, only some of which have been explored in the scholarship.

© The Author(s), under exclusive license to Springer Nature
Switzerland AG 2022
K. Kennedy, *Frank Herbert's* Dune, Palgrave Science Fiction and
Fantasy: A New Canon,
https://doi.org/10.1007/978-3-031-13935-2_7

World-building is an emerging area of study well-suited to *Dune* and the fictional world it and its sequels have created. World-building theory looks at characteristics of imagined worlds, particularly those in science fiction and fantasy. It examines how authors create immersive worlds that readers want to explore, how they give the illusion that a fantastical place could really exist. Considered by many to represent the pinnacle of world-building in science fiction, *Dune* has a memorable desert planet with giant sandworms but also much more than that. Herbert creates a clash of cultures through the depiction of the Atreides family and the Fremen, and he uses names as a key part of his strategy. Thus, Jessica and Paul Atreides have names associated with Western culture, mythology, and Christianity, and the Fremen use names derived from Arabic and Islam [1]. The invention of the substance of spice is another tool of world-building. By centering the universe on this one precious resource, found only in a desert environment closely resembling that of the Middle East, Herbert makes crucial connections with real-world analogies in the spice trade and oil industry and focuses our attention on ecological disruptions at an individual and societal level [2]. Drawing on his understanding of social sciences such as psychology, linguistics, and sociology, he develops a world focused more on humans than technology [3]. All of these elements combine to make the world seem familiar yet new and engage our attention in the first and subsequent readings.

Materials outside of the main storyline also can be studied for the contribution they make to the development of the world. Herbert's use of epigraphs that are excerpts from the fictional writings of Princess Irulan provides a different feel to the book than if he had merely included the main story. Her first epigraph opens *Dune* in the epic tradition by identifying the hero, the time of the story's events, and the location [4, p. 136]. Irulan thus crafts an image of Paul as a mythic, legendary figure from the beginning. She uses the name Muad'Dib, which he will not take on for many chapters. We have the sense that everything has already happened. Through the epigraphs, Herbert foreshadows the events of the chapter and alters readers' perspectives on them. We learn about people before we see them, just as Paul does with his visions. We gain insights into palace life before meeting the Emperor and his court at the end of the book. Through the epigraphs, Irulan's knowledge plays against our ignorance until we finish each chapter [5, p. 89]. There are also four appendices that provide additional context and historical explanations for character and group behaviors: The Ecology of Dune, The Religion of Dune, Report on Bene

Gesserit Motives and Purposes, and The Almanak en-Ashraf (Selected Excerpts of the Noble Houses). Following them is a glossary that acknowledges there are many unfamiliar terms in the book and proposes to help increase understanding by providing short definitions. Finally, there are cartographic notes and a map that help us visualize what the author had in mind for his world. These extra features assist with the world-building by giving us the sense that the world extends beyond the time and events described within, and that Dune could be a real planet.

The frequent sprinkling of words from languages other than English offers fruitful opportunities for linguistic analysis. As the bestselling science fiction novel, *Dune* has been translated into many non-English languages and offers a worthwhile case for translation studies. Translators are presented with numerous challenges: they must determine how to translate invented terms such as crysknife or baliset—an issue with many translations of science fiction—but they must also look at Herbert's complex use of loanwords, or words that already are taken directly from other languages such as Arabic. Loanwords present a complication in that they do not always line up exactly with their real-life meaning, since Herbert uses them to create a certain context and color for his imagined world [6, p. 183]. For example, the Arabic names Ikhwan (fraternity) and Bedouin (Arabic-speaking nomadic peoples of Middle Eastern deserts) are turned into the loanwords 'Ichwan Bedwine,' defined in *Dune* as the brotherhood of all Fremen. A French translation study has found differences in spelling, capitalization, and use of hyphens when Arabic loanwords in *Dune* have been translated [6, p. 193]. El-Sayal becomes El sayal, and baklawa becomes baklava, for instance. This signals the flexibility and creativity that translators employ to try to keep the foreign feel of Arabic while adapting some of the words to suit readers of non-English languages.

Looking at *Dune* through a postcolonial lens raises questions about the characterization of the Fremen and their position as a colonized and marginalized people on Arrakis. The Fremen are essential to the storyline and the larger ecological messages underpinning the book. They are often overlooked in favor of a focus on Paul or dismissed as victims of religious manipulation. Yet they are constructed with a rich base from a variety of real-world cultures and offer more than a simple black-and-white case of oppressed peoples. Herbert is not faultless in his depiction, but his relationships with friends from the Native American Quileute community in Washington had a noticeable impact on his understanding and sympathy toward the plight of marginalized groups [7]. Herbert does more than copy the Lawrence of Arabia story in his treatment of the locals [8]. The Fremen merit a more comprehensive study that covers the characterization of their past, their struggles, their triumphs, and their approach to their desert habitat.

For those who enjoy exploring the meaning of imagery and symbols in literature, *Dune* contains a wealth of potential. Sand is probably the most obvious image. Sand dunes are echoed in the book's title and appear on most book covers. Key events revolve around this prominent feature of the desert environment, including characters having to walk on the sand without attracting sandworms, and Paul coming to greater awareness while staying in the stilltent buried in the sand with his mother on their flight into the desert. Sand is traditionally linked with the passage of time, as in hourglasses, and the sense of an uncountable vastness. In the book, it is bound up with the images of the sandworm and spice. The sandworm can symbolize divine energy and as the 'maker' suggests eternity [9, p. 132]. Spice also has connections with transcendence and the eternal, as well as prophecy and history due to its role in unlocking prescient powers [9, p. 132]. Water is another important image. The arid desert environment emphasizes the importance of this life-sustaining substance, as does the characterization of the Fremen. Their culture is centered on water: the Water of Life ceremony illustrates their special relationship with spice-infused liquid, their courtship rituals involve water rings, and spitting or shedding tears for the dead marks the ultimate gift of the body's moisture. Water is also associated with the flow of time as well as spiritual dimensions [9, p. 131]. Other types of imagery include religious images, archetypal images, fractal images, Gothic symbols, and the blue eyes of those addicted to spice.

A psychological reading of *Dune* might look at Freudian or Jungian themes and imagery. There are several examples of Paul being 'birthed' into a new environment. For instance, he goes from the wet world of Caladan to the desert world of Dune [10, p. 18]. He also experiences a birth upon emerging from the stilltent with a fuller sense of his identity. This is when he discovers that the Baron is his maternal grandfather, which is a situation ripe for Freudian analysis. Oedipal conflict can be seen in Paul's relationship with his father and mother, with potential incest taboos, unconscious guilt, and fear of the feminine shaping the young hero's life [11, p. 151]. There are also other examples of familial conflict: Feyd-Rautha tries to poison his uncle, the Baron, Irulan suspects that her father has tried to murder her and her mother and sisters, and Alia succeeds in killing the Baron just as he is attempting to kill her [11, p. 152]. Reverend Mother Mohiam's mysterious black box of pain may be viewed as an image of castration anxiety, especially since she admits that she wanted Paul to fail and subjected him to a higher level than anyone else had withstood [11, p. 154]. Phallic imagery includes sandworms and Paul's test of riding them as a passage to manhood. In terms of Jungian concepts, there is a parallel between the collective unconscious and the Bene Gesserit's ancestral memory. There are also Jungian archetypes and character development using concepts of extroversion–introversion, thinking–feeling, and sensing–intuition [12, p. 11]. The way the Voice works on the level of people's unconscious may also be viewed from a psychological perspective.

A comparative literary approach takes into consideration other works of science fiction that are either similar to or juxtaposed with *Dune*. Some view *Dune* as a critical response to Isaac Asimov's epic *Foundation* trilogy (1951–1953), which features a group of psychohistorians who seek to shape the future through scientific predictions and mathematical calculations. In this view, Herbert has replaced Hari Seldon and his mathematics with Paul Muad'Dib and his wild unconscious, and order and civilization with anarchy and nature [5, p. 79]. Herbert turns the male scientists into the female Bene Gesserit and exposes the shortcomings of their attempt to control the future through their breeding program. Both deal with the theme of the decline of a dying empire and the emergence of a new, vital population [13, p. 269]. There is a similar move from a place representing a stagnant civilization to a primitive world, which becomes the launching point for a new and better civilization [14, p. 151]. While in *Foundation* missionaries are sent to create a religion of science, in *Dune* Bene Gesserit missionaries are sent to insert new dogma for exploitation by future Bene Gesserit. Yet both stories present religion as a construct designed to pave the way for outsiders to gain power [14, p. 151]. They also offer a type of future prediction or prescience to characters in order to explore how knowledge of what is ahead affects humanity, for better or worse [14, p. 152].

Another approach is to compare *Dune* with classical works and the epic tradition. Epics in the Western tradition include Homer's *Iliad* and *Odyssey* and John Milton's *Paradise Lost* (1667), all of which have had significant and long-lasting impacts on literature. *Dune* has many of the characteristics associated with epics: it concerns itself with great events, features great figures, and has military battles like those in heroic poetry [15, pp. 205–206]. It is centered on Paul as a heroic man who has superior abilities, like Odysseus or Achilles, and whose actions have large-scale consequences that alter history [4, pp. 132–133]. The final showdown includes ships from throughout the Imperium orbiting the planet, elevating the confrontation to epic heights. *Dune* also relies heavily on the conventions around prophets and prophecies to create a strong sense of epic suspense and destiny [15, p. 206]. Paul represents the realization of the Bene Gesserit's plan to produce the Kwisatz Haderach, a figure who can look into the past and the future like Tiresias, the blind prophet from Greek mythology. Paul's prescient visions are similar to the godly prophecies in classical epics, but remain subjective and so leave open the possibility for events to occur differently than how he predicts they will [15, pp. 210–211]. The many parallels with the epic tradition in the book's characters and events provide the kind of depth that helps elevate the book's literary status.

A posthumanist study of *Dune* might look at the different aspects of human advancement and augmentation and how they relate to the evolution of humanity. Posthumanism in science fiction can refer to changes made to the human body, a world not centered on humans, or the consequences of the march toward a future dominated by technoscientific control [16]. *Dune* is somewhat unusual in that Herbert specifically sets up a historical context in which advanced technology has been banned after the Butlerian Jihad. This results in human enhancement largely coming from rigorous training or the ingesting of spice, or a combination of both. Most characters have some level of special training or development, whether they be Mentats, fighters, doctors, or scientists. We see Paul curious about the deformation and mutation of Guild navigators before his own transformation into a spice-fueled prescient being. We see Jessica expand her psyche to include a line of female ancestors, and her unborn daughter taken along for the ride and also turned into a Reverend Mother. Although these changes are fantastical, they raise questions about the adaptations or special abilities humans may take on in the future.

From a philosophical perspective, *Dune* offers rich material for exploration. Characters' ability to see into the future raises questions about the nature of free will and determinism. On the one hand, Paul seems to have visions of possible futures rather than one predetermined future. This avoids the paradox of foreknowledge, in which someone can see the future but cannot change it [17, p. 37]. On the other hand, Paul is unable to avoid the coming jihad, much as he might try, which suggests that his ability to choose a different future is limited. The book is also open to questions of ethics. We might consider the ethics of the Kynes' environmental project, the Bene Gesserit's eugenics-driven breeding program, Paul and Jessica's exploitation of the Missionaria Protectiva, or the Fremen's moral code. Herbert avoids creating situations and behaviors that are clearly good or bad, forcing us to come to our own conclusions. It is also possible to use various philosophers' theories as a lens to examine the book. For instance, Friedrich Nietzsche's concept of the Overman and the will to power can be applied to Paul's character [18, 19]. René Descartes' concept of the separation between mind and body and Simone de Beauvoir's refutation of such dualistic thinking can be used to compare the training of the Bene Gesserit and the Mentats [20]. Existential philosophies from Martin Heidegger and Karl Jaspers offer pathways to understanding the nature of human existence as presented in the book. With *Dune* so focused on the nature of humans, it provides many avenues for philosophical discovery and analysis.

Frank Herbert's *Dune* is a masterwork of science fiction with a body of scholarship that has really only scratched the surface of its many layers. Its deceptively simple storyline rests on a mountain of historical and philosophical contexts and influences that provide a richness of development which continues to attract readers. Its ambiguity and openness to multiple interpretations make it ripe for new critical perspectives and debates. And its complexity and themes have helped turn it into a classic, a work of literature that stands poised to continue appealing to audiences into the future.

References

1. Kennedy, Kara. "Epic World-Building: Names and Cultures in *Dune*." *Names*, vol. 64, no. 2, 2016, pp. 99–108.
2. Kennedy, Kara. "Spice and Ecology in Herbert's *Dune*: Altering the Mind and the Planet." *Science Fiction Studies*, vol. 48, no. 3, 2021, pp. 444–461.
3. Kennedy, Kara. "The Softer Side of *Dune*: The Impact of the Social Sciences on World-Building." *Exploring Imaginary Worlds: Essays on Media, Structure, and Subcreation*, edited by Mark J.P. Wolf, Routledge, 2020, pp. 159–174.
4. Collings, Michael R. "The Epic of *Dune*: Epic Traditions in Modern Science Fiction." *Aspects of Fantasy: Selected Essays from the Second International Conference on the Fantastic in Literature and Film*, edited by William Coyle, Greenwood Press, 1986, pp. 131–139.

5. Manlove, C.N. "Frank Herbert, *Dune* (1965)." *Science Fiction: Ten Explorations*. Macmillan Press, 1986, pp. 79–99.
6. Ray, Alice. "The Translation of *Dune*: An Encounter of Languages." *Contacts and Contrasts in Educational Contexts and Translation*, edited by Barbara Lewandowska-Tomaszczyk, Springer, 2019, pp. 183–194.
7. Immerwahr, Daniel. "The Quileute *Dune*: Frank Herbert, Indigeneity, and Empire." *Journal of American Studies*, vol. 56, no. 2, 2022, pp. 191–216.
8. Kennedy, Kara. "Lawrence of Arabia, Paul Atreides, and the Roots of Frank Herbert's Dune." *Tor.com*, 2 June 2021. https://www.tor.com/2021/06/02/lawrence-of-arabia-paul-atreides-and-the-roots-of-frank-herberts-dune/
9. Ower, John. "Idea and Imagery in Herbert's *Dune*." *Extrapolation*, vol. 15, no. 2, 1974, pp. 129–139.
10. Parkinson, Robert C. "*Dune* – An Unfinished Tetralogy." *Extrapolation*, vol. 13, no. 1, 1971, pp. 16–24.
11. McLean, Susan. "A Psychological Approach to Fantasy in the *Dune* Series." *Extrapolation*, vol. 23, no. 2, 1982, pp. 150–158.
12. Touponce, William. *Frank Herbert*. Twayne Publishers, 1988.
13. DiTommaso, Lorenzo. "The Articulation of Imperial Decadence and Decline in Epic Science Fiction." *Extrapolation*, vol. 48, no. 2, 2007, pp. 267–291.
14. Grigsby, John L. "Asimov's 'Foundation' Trilogy and Herbert's 'Dune' Trilogy: A Vision Reversed." *Science Fiction Studies*, vol. 8, no. 2, 1981, pp. 149–155.
15. Cirasa, Robert. "An Epic Impression: Suspense and Prophetic Conventions in the Classical Epics and Frank Herbert's *Dune*." *Classical and Modern Literature*, vol. 4, 1984, pp. 195–213.
16. Vint, Sherryl. "Science Fiction and Posthumanism." *Critical Posthumanism*, 24 May 2016. https://criticalposthumanism.net/science-fiction/
17. Gates-Scovelle, Sam. "Curse of the Golden Path." *Dune and Philosophy: Weirding Way of the Mentat*, edited by Jeffery Nicholas, Open Court, 2011, pp. 37–49.
18. Jackson, Roy. "Paul Atreides the Nietzschean Hero." *Dune and Philosophy: Weirding Way of the Mentat*, edited by Jeffery Nicholas, Open Court, 2011, pp. 177–187.
19. Pearson, Brook W.R. "Friedrich Nietzsche Goes to Space." *Dune and Philosophy: Weirding Way of the Mentat*, edited by Jeffery Nicholas, Open Court, 2011, pp. 189–205.
20. Kennedy, Kara. *Women's Agency in the* Dune *Universe: Tracing Women's Liberation through Science Fiction*. Palgrave Macmillan, 2021.

Bibliography

Ali, R. "Beside the Sand Dunes: Arab Futurism, Faith, and the Fremen of Dune." *Discovering Dune: Essays on Frank Herbert's Epic Saga*, edited by Dominic J. Nardi and N. Trevor Brierly, McFarland, forthcoming.

Allen, David L. *Cliffs Notes on Herbert's Dune and Other Works*. Cliffs Notes, 1975.

Altinkaya, Galipcan, and Mehmet Kuyurtar. "Lessons from Islamic Philosophy on the Politics of Paul Atreides." *Dune and Philosophy: Minds, Monads, and Muad'Dib*, edited by Kevin S. Decker, Wiley-Blackwell, forthcoming.

Anderson, Daniel Gustav. "Critical Bioregionalist Method in Dune: A Position Paper." *The Bioregional Imagination: Literature, Ecology, and Place*, edited by Cheryll Glotfelty, Karla Armbruster, and Tom Lynch, University of Georgia Press, 2012, pp. 226–242.

Asher-Perrin, Emmet. "Why It's Important to Consider Whether *Dune* Is a White Savior Narrative." *Tor.com*, 6 Mar. 2019. https://www.tor.com/2019/03/06/why-its-important-to-consider-whether-dune-is-a-white-savior-narrative/.

Baade, Björnstjern. "The Law of Frank Herbert's *Dune*: Legal Culture between Cynicism, Earnestness and Futility." *Law & Literature*, 2022, pp. 1–31.

Barbour, Douglas. "Occasional Thoughts on Frank Herbert's *Dune* Sequence." *The Australian Science Fiction Review*, vol. 3, no. 6 / vol. 4, no. 1, 1988 / 1989, pp. 10–13.

Bein, Steve. "That Which Does Not Kill Me Makes Me Shai-Hulud: Self-Overcoming in Nietzsche, Hinduism, and *Dune*." *Dune and Philosophy: Minds, Monads, and Muad'Dib*, edited by Kevin S. Decker, Wiley-Blackwell, forthcoming.

Brierly, N. Trevor. "'A critical moment': The O.C. Bible in the Awakening of Paul Atreides." *Discovering Dune: Essays on Frank Herbert's Epic Saga*, edited by Dominic J. Nardi and N. Trevor Brierly, McFarland, forthcoming.

Butkus, Matthew A. "A Universe of Bastards." *Dune and Philosophy: Weirding Way of the Mentat*, edited by Jeffery Nicholas, Open Court, 2011, pp. 75–87.

Carroll, Jordan S. "Race Consciousness: Fascism and Frank Herbert's 'Dune.'" *Los Angeles Review of Books*, 19 Nov. 2020. https://lareviewofbooks.org/article/race-consciousness-fascism-and-frank-herberts-dune/.

Christensen, Joel P. "Time and Self-Referentiality in the *Iliad* and Frank Herbert's *Dune*." *Classical Traditions in Science Fiction*, edited by B. M. Rogers and B. E. Stevens, Oxford University Press, 2015, pp. 161–175.

Ciocchetti, Christopher. "Power Mongers and Worm Riders." *Dune and Philosophy: Weirding Way of the Mentat*, edited by Jeffery Nicholas, Open Court, 2011, pp. 91–101.

Cirasa, Robert. "An Epic Impression: Suspense and Prophetic Conventions in the Classical Epics and Frank Herbert's *Dune*." *Classical and Modern Literature*, vol. 4, 1984, pp. 195–213.

Collings, Michael R. "The Epic of *Dune*: Epic Traditions in Modern Science Fiction." *Aspects of Fantasy: Selected Essays from the Second International Conference on the Fantastic in Literature and Film*, edited by William Coyle, Greenwood Press, 1986, pp. 131–139.

Collins, Will. "The Secret History of Dune." *Los Angeles Review of Books*, 16 Sept. 2017. https://lareviewofbooks.org/article/the-secret-history-of-dune.

Crippen, Matthew. "Psychological Expanses of *Dune*: Indigenous Philosophy, Americana and Existentialism." *Dune and Philosophy: Minds, Monads, and Muad'Dib*, edited by Kevin S. Decker, Wiley-Blackwell, forthcoming.

Csori, Csilla. "Memory (and the Tleilaxu) Makes the Man." *The Science of Dune: An Unauthorized Exploration into the Real Science Behind Frank Herbert's Fictional Universe*, edited by Kevin R. Grazier, BenBella Books, 2008a, pp. 167–176.

Csori, Csilla. "Prescience and Prophecy." *The Science of Dune: An Unauthorized Exploration into the Real Science Behind Frank Herbert's Fictional Universe*, edited by Kevin R. Grazier, BenBella Books, 2008b, pp. 111–126.

Daniels, Joseph M. *The Stars and Planets of Frank Herbert's* Dune*: A Gazetteer*. 1999.

Dawson, Allan Charles, and Ismael Vaccaro. "Territorializing Arrakis: Competing for Water and Melange at the Edge of the Galactic Empire – Between Desert Gatherers and the Spacefaring." *Handbook on Space, Place and Law*, edited by Robyn Bartel and Jennifer Carter, Edward Elgar Publishing, 2021, pp. 293–303.

Decker, Kevin S. "'Thatched Cottages at Cordeville': Hegel, Heidegger and the Death of Art in *Dune*." *Dune and Philosophy: Minds, Monads, and Muad'Dib*, edited by Kevin S. Decker, Wiley-Blackwell, forthcoming.

DiPasquale, Willow Wilson. "Shifting Sands: Heroes, Power, and the Environment in the Dune Saga." *Discovering Dune: Essays on Frank Herbert's Epic Saga*, edited by Dominic J. Nardi and N. Trevor Brierly, McFarland, forthcoming.
DiTommaso, Lorenzo. "The Articulation of Imperial Decadence and Decline in Epic Science Fiction." *Extrapolation*, vol. 48, no. 2, 2007, pp. 267–291.
DiTommaso, Lorenzo. "History and Historical Effect in Frank Herbert's 'Dune.'" *Science Fiction Studies*, vol. 19, no. 3, 1992, pp. 311–325.
Dragomir, Alexandru. "'Less Than a God, More than a Man': Is It Morally Wrong to Make a Kwisatz Haderach?" *Dune and Philosophy: Minds, Monads, and Muad'Dib*, edited by Kevin S. Decker, Wiley-Blackwell, forthcoming.
Durrani, Haris. "The Muslimness of *Dune*: A Close Reading of 'Appendix II: The Religion of Dune.'" *Tor.com*, 18 Oct. 2021. https://www.tor.com/2021/10/18/the-muslimness-of-dune-a-close-reading-of-appendix-ii-the-religion-of-dune/.
Elgin, Don D. "Frank Herbert." *The Comedy of the Fantastic: Ecological Perspectives on the Fantasy Novel*, Greenwood Press, 1985, pp. 125–152.
Ellis, R. J. "Frank Herbert's *Dune* and the Discourse of Apocalyptic Ecologism in the United States." *Science Fiction Roots and Branches: Contemporary Critical Approaches*, edited by Rhys Garnett and R. J. Ellis, Macmillan Press, 1990, pp. 104–124.
Erman, Eva, and Niklas Möller. "What's Wrong with Politics in the Duniverse?" *Dune and Philosophy: Weirding Way of the Mentat*, edited by Jeffery Nicholas, Open Court, 2011, pp. 61–73.
Farnsworth, Alex, Michael Farnsworth, and Sebastian Steinig. "Dune: We Simulated the Desert Planet of Arrakis to See If Humans Could Survive There." *The Conversation*, 26 Oct. 2021. https://theconversation.com/dune-we-simulated-the-desert-planet-of-arrakis-to-see-if-humans-could-survive-there-170181.
Ferner, Adam. "Memories Are Made of Spice." *Dune and Philosophy: Weirding Way of the Mentat*, edited by Jeffery Nicholas, Open Court, 2011, pp. 161–174.
Field, Gemma. "Dune Rehabilitation in Progress." *Journal of Literary Studies*, vol. 34, no. 3, 2018, pp. 123–137.
Field, Sandy. "Evolution by Any Means on Dune." *The Science of Dune: An Unauthorized Exploration into the Real Science Behind Frank Herbert's Fictional Universe*, edited by Kevin R. Grazier, BenBella Books, 2008, pp. 67–82.
Fjellman, Stephen M. "Prescience and Power: 'God Emperor of Dune' and the Intellectuals." *Science Fiction Studies*, vol. 13, no. 1, 1986, pp. 50–63.
Forsythe, Sam. "The Mind at War: Conflict and Cognition in Frank Herbert's *Dune*." *Dune and Philosophy: Minds, Monads, and Muad'Dib*, edited by Kevin S. Decker, Wiley-Blackwell, forthcoming.
Freitas, Joana Gaspar de. "*Dune*(s): Fiction, History, and Science on the Oregon Coast." *The Anthropocene Review*, 2021, pp. 1–9.

Gates-Scovelle, Sam. "Curse of the Golden Path." *Dune and Philosophy: Weirding Way of the Mentat*, edited by Jeffery Nicholas, Open Court, 2011a, pp. 37–49.
Gates-Scovelle, Sam. "Son of the Curse of the Golden Path." *Dune and Philosophy: Weirding Way of the Mentat*, edited by Jeffery Nicholas, Open Court, 2011b, pp. 207–217.
Gates-Scovelle, Sam, and Stephanie Semler. "A Ghola of a Chance." *Dune and Philosophy: Weirding Way of the Mentat*, edited by Jeffery Nicholas, Open Court, 2011, pp. 131–148.
Gaylard, Gerald. "Postcolonialism and the Transhistorical in *Dune*." *Foundation*, vol. 37, no. 104, 2008, pp. 88–101.
Gaylard, Gerald. "Postcolonial Science Fiction: The Desert Planet." *Science Fiction, Imperialism, and the Third World: Essays on Postcolonial Literature and Film*, edited by Ericka Hoagland and Reema Sarwal, McFarland, 2010, pp. 21–36.
Goldberg, Nathaniel. "The Sands of Time: *Dune* and the Philosophy of Time." *Discovering Dune: Essays on Frank Herbert's Epic Saga*, edited by Dominic J. Nardi and N. Trevor Brierly, McFarland, forthcoming.
Gough, Noel. "Speculative Fictions for Understanding Global Change Environments, Two Thought Experiments." *Managing Global Transitions*, vol. 1, no. 1, 2003, pp. 5–27.
Grazier, Kevin R. "Cosmic Origami: Folded Space and FTL in the Duniverse." *The Science of Dune: An Unauthorized Exploration into the Real Science Behind Frank Herbert's Fictional Universe*, edited by Kevin R. Grazier, BenBella Books, 2008a, pp. 177–206.
Grazier, Kevin R. "Introduction." *The Science of Dune: An Unauthorized Exploration into the Real Science Behind Frank Herbert's Fictional Universe*, edited by Kevin R. Grazier, BenBella Books, 2008b, pp. vii–ix.
Grazier, Kevin R. "The Real Stars of Dune." *The Science of Dune: An Unauthorized Exploration into the Real Science Behind Frank Herbert's Fictional Universe*, edited by Kevin R. Grazier, BenBella Books, 2008c, pp. 89–110.
Grigsby, John L. "Asimov's 'Foundation' Trilogy and Herbert's 'Dune' Trilogy: A Vision Reversed." *Science Fiction Studies*, vol. 8, no. 2, 1981, pp. 149–155.
Grigsby, John L. "Herbert's Reversal of Asimov's Vision Reassessed: 'Foundation's Edge' and 'God Emperor of Dune.'" *Science Fiction Studies*, vol. 11, no. 33, 1984, pp. 174–180.
Hand, Jack. "The Traditionalism of Women's Roles in Frank Herbert's *Dune*." *Extrapolation*, vol. 26, no. 1, 1985, pp. 24–28.
Hart, Carol. "The Black Hole of Pain." *The Science of Dune: An Unauthorized Exploration into the Real Science Behind Frank Herbert's Fictional Universe*, edited by Kevin R. Grazier, BenBella Books, 2008a, pp. 143–150.
Hart, Carol. "From Silver Fox to Kwisatz Haderach: The Possibilities of Selective Breeding Programs." *The Science of Dune: An Unauthorized Exploration into*

the Real Science Behind Frank Herbert's Fictional Universe, edited by Kevin R. Grazier, BenBella Books, 2008b, pp. 59–66.
Hart, Carol. "Melange." *The Science of Dune: An Unauthorized Exploration into the Real Science Behind Frank Herbert's Fictional Universe*, edited by Kevin R. Grazier, BenBella Books, 2008c, pp. 1–20.
Hechtel, Sibyelle. "The Biology of the Sandworm." *The Science of Dune: An Unauthorized Exploration into the Real Science Behind Frank Herbert's Fictional Universe*, edited by Kevin R. Grazier, BenBella Books, 2008, pp. 29–48.
Herbert, Brian. *Dreamer of Dune: The Biography of Frank Herbert*. Tom Doherty Associates, 2003.
Herbert, Frank. *Maker of Dune*, edited by Tim O'Reilly, Berkley Books, 1987.
Herbert, Frank and Beverly. Interview by Willis E. McNelly. 3 Feb. 1969.
Herman, Peter. "The Blackness of Liet-Kynes: Reading Frank Herbert's *Dune* Through James Cone." *Religions*, vol. 9, no. 9, 2018, pp. 281–290.
Higgins, David M. "Psychic Decolonization in 1960s Science Fiction." *Science Fiction Studies*, vol. 40, no. 2, 2013, pp. 228–245.
Hillman, Luke. "The Spice of Life: Hedonism and Nozick in the *Dune* Universe." *Dune and Philosophy: Minds, Monads, and Muad'Dib*, edited by Kevin S. Decker, Wiley-Blackwell, forthcoming.
Hoberek, Andrew. "*Dune*, the Middle Class and Post-1960 U.S. Foreign Policy." *American Literature and Culture in an Age of Cold War: A Critical Reassessment*, edited by Daniel Grausam and Steven Belletto, Iowa University Press, 2012, pp. 85–108.
Hones, Sheila. "The Geosophical Structure of Frank Herbert's *Dune*." *Keisen Jogakuen College Bulletin*, 1990, no. 2, pp. 1–31.
Houot, A.M. "Spiritual Realm Adaptation: Arrakeen Spice, Terrestrial Psychedelics, and Technique." *Dune and Philosophy: Minds, Monads, and Muad'Dib*, edited by Kevin S. Decker, Wiley-Blackwell, forthcoming.
Immerwahr, Daniel. "Heresies of 'Dune.'" *Los Angeles Review of Books*, 19 Nov. 2020. https://www.lareviewofbooks.org/article/heresies-of-dune/.
Immerwahr, Daniel. "The Quileute *Dune*: Frank Herbert, Indigeneity, and Empire." *Journal of American Studies*, vol. 56, no. 2, 2022, pp. 191–216.
Irvin, Alan. "Time versus History: A Conflict Central to Herbert's *Dune*." *Dune and Philosophy: Minds, Monads, and Muad'Dib*, edited by Kevin S. Decker, Wiley-Blackwell, forthcoming.
Jackson, Roy. "Paul Atreides the Nietzschean Hero." *Dune and Philosophy: Weirding Way of the Mentat*, edited by Jeffery Nicholas, Open Court, 2011, pp. 177–187.
Jacob, Frank. "Jihad in Outer Space: The Orientalist Semiotics of Frank Herbert's *Dune* and the Image of Lawrence of Arabia." *War in Film: Semiotics and Conflict Related Sign Constructions on the Screen*, Büchner-Verlag, 2022a, pp. 51–96.

Jacob, Frank. *The Orientalist Semiotics of Dune: Religious and Historical References within Frank Herbert's Universe*. Büchner-Verlag, 2022b.

Kennedy, Kara. "Epic World-Building: Names and Cultures in *Dune*." *Names*, vol. 64, no. 2, 2016, pp. 99–108.

Kennedy, Kara. "Frank Herbert, the Bene Gesserit, and the Complexity of Women in the World of *Dune*." *Tor.com*, 8 Sept. 2021a. https://www.tor.com/2021/09/08/frank-herbert-the-bene-gesserit-and-the-complexity-of-women-in-the-world-of-dune/.

Kennedy, Kara. "Lawrence of Arabia, Paul Atreides, and the Roots of Frank Herbert's *Dune*." *Tor.com*, 2 Jun. 2021b. https://www.tor.com/2021/06/02/lawrence-of-arabia-paul-atreides-and-the-roots-of-frank-herberts-dune/.

Kennedy, Kara. "Liberating Women's Bodies: Feminist Philosophy and the Bene Gesserit of *Dune*." *Dune and Philosophy: Minds, Monads, and Muad'Dib*, edited by Kevin S. Decker, Wiley-Blackwell, forthcoming.

Kennedy, Kara. "The Softer Side of *Dune*: The Impact of the Social Sciences on World-Building." *Exploring Imaginary Worlds: Essays on Media, Structure, and Subcreation*, edited by Mark J.P. Wolf, Routledge, 2020, pp. 159–174.

Kennedy, Kara. "Spice and Ecology in Herbert's *Dune*: Altering the Mind and the Planet." *Science Fiction Studies*, vol. 48, no. 3, 2021c, pp. 444–461.

Kennedy, Kara. *Women's Agency in the Dune Universe: Tracing Women's Liberation through Science Fiction*. Palgrave Macmillan, 2021d.

Kokkonen, Tomi, Ilmari Hirvonen, and Matti Mäkikangas. "'Thou Shalt Make a Human Mind in the Likeness of a Machine': Imitation, Thinking Machines and Mentats." *Dune and Philosophy: Minds, Monads, and Muad'Dib*, edited by Kevin S. Decker, Wiley-Blackwell, forthcoming.

Kratz, Veronika. "Frank Herbert's Ecology, Oregon's Dunes, and the Postwar Science of Desert Reclamation." *ISLE: Interdisciplinary Studies in Literature and Environment*, 2021, pp. 1–20.

Kucera, Paul Q. "Listening to Ourselves: Herbert's *Dune*, 'the Voice,' and Performing the Absolute." *Extrapolation*, vol. 42, no. 3, 2001, pp. 232–245.

Kunzru, Hari. "*Dune*, 50 Years On: How a Science Fiction Novel Changed the World." *The Guardian*, 3 Jul. 2015. https://www.theguardian.com/books/2015/jul/03/dune-50-years-on-science-fiction-novel-world.

Lau, Maximilian. "Frank Herbert's Byzantium: Medieval-Futurism and the Princess Historians Irulan and Anna Komnene." *Discovering Dune: Essays on Frank Herbert's Epic Saga*, edited by Dominic J. Nardi and N. Trevor Brierly, McFarland, forthcoming.

Lawrence, David M. "The Shade of Uliet: Musings on the Ecology of *Dune*." *The Science of Dune: An Unauthorized Exploration into the Real Science Behind Frank Herbert's Fictional Universe*, edited by Kevin R. Grazier, BenBella Books, 2008, pp. 217–232.

Leonard, Andrew. "To Save California, Read 'Dune.'" *Nautilus*, 4 Jun. 2015. https://nautil.us/issue/25/water/to-save-california-read-dune.

List, Julia. "'Call me a Protestant': Liberal Christianity, Individualism, and the Messiah in *Stranger in a Strange Land*, *Dune*, and *Lord of Light*." *Science Fiction Studies*, vol. 36, no. 1, 2009, pp. 21–47.

Littmann, Greg. "Just What Do You Do with the Entire Human Race Anyway?" *Dune and Philosophy: Weirding Way of the Mentat*, edited by Jeffery Nicholas, Open Court, 2011, pp. 103–119.

Littmann, Greg. "Messiahs, Jihads and God Emperors: Should Humanity Just Give up Religion?" *Dune and Philosophy: Minds, Monads, and Muad'Dib*, edited by Kevin S. Decker, Wiley-Blackwell, forthcoming-a.

Littmann, Greg. "Should the Bene Gesserit Be in Charge?" *Dune and Philosophy: Minds, Monads, and Muad'Dib*, edited by Kevin S. Decker, Wiley-Blackwell, forthcoming-b.

Lorenz, Ralph D. "The Dunes of Dune: The Planetology of Arrakis." *The Science of Dune: An Unauthorized Exploration into the Real Science Behind Frank Herbert's Fictional Universe*, edited by Kevin R. Grazier, BenBella Books, 2008, pp. 49–58.

Lund, Kristian. "Wiping Finite Answers from an Infinite Universe." *Dune and Philosophy: Weirding Way of the Mentat*, edited by Jeffery Nicholas, Open Court, 2011, pp. 149–160.

Mack, Robert L. "Voice Lessons: The Seductive Appeal of Vocal Control in Frank Herbert's *Dune*." *Journal of the Fantastic in the Arts*, vol. 22, no. 1, 2011, pp. 39–59.

Manlove, C.N. "Frank Herbert, *Dune* (1965)." *Science Fiction: Ten Explorations*. Macmillan Press, 1986, pp. 79–99.

McLean, Susan. "A Psychological Approach to Fantasy in the *Dune* Series." *Extrapolation*, vol. 23, no. 2, 1982, pp. 150–158.

McLean, Susan. "A Question of Balance: Death and Immortality in Frank Herbert's Dune Series." *Death and the Serpent*, edited by Carl Yoke, Greenwood Press, 1985, pp. 145–152.

McNelly, Willis E., and Timothy O'Reilly. "*Dune*." *Survey of Science Fiction Literature*, vol. 2, edited by Frank N. Magill, Salem Press, 1979, pp. 647–658.

McReynolds, Leigha High. "Locations of Deviance: A Eugenics Reading of Dune." *Discovering Dune: Essays on Frank Herbert's Epic Saga*, edited by Dominic J. Nardi and N. Trevor Brierly, McFarland, forthcoming.

Melançon, Louis. "Shifting Sand, Shifting Balance." *Dune and Philosophy: Weirding Way of the Mentat*, edited by Jeffery Nicholas, Open Court, 2011, pp. 27–35.

Mellamphy, Nandita Biswas. "Terra-&-Terror Ecology: Secrets from the Arrakeen Underground." *Design Ecologies*, vol. 3, no. 1, 2013, pp. 66–91.

Michaud, Jon. "'Dune' Endures." *The New Yorker*, 12 July 2013. https://www.newyorker.com/books/page-turner/dune-endures.
Miller, David. *Frank Herbert*. Starmont House, 1980.
Miller, Miriam Youngerman. "Women of *Dune*: Frank Herbert as Social Reactionary?" *Women Worldwalkers: New Dimensions of Science Fiction and Fantasy*, edited by Jane B. Weedman, Texas Tech University Press, 1985, pp. 181–192.
Mills, Ethan. "The Golden Path and Multicultural Meanings of Life." *Dune and Philosophy: Minds, Monads, and Muad'Dib*, edited by Kevin S. Decker, Wiley-Blackwell, forthcoming
Minowitz, Peter. "Prince versus Prophet: Machiavellianism in Frank Herbert's *Dune* Epic." *Political Science Fiction*, edited by Donald M. Hassler and Clyde Wilcox, University of South Carolina Press, 1996, pp. 124–147.
Mohamed, Hussain Rafi. "Ecological Niche: Frank Herbert 1920–1986. A Personal Recollection of the Dune Books of Frank Herbert." *Vector*, vol. 42, no. 131, 1986, p. 11.
Morton, Timothy. "Imperial Measures: *Dune*, Ecology and Romantic Consumerism." *Romanticism On the Net*, no. 21, 2001. https://id.erudit.org/iderudit/005966ar.
Mulcahy, Kevin. "*The Prince* on Arrakis: Frank Herbert's Dialogue with Machiavelli." *Extrapolation*, vol. 37, no. 1, 1996, pp. 22–36.
Nardi, Dominic J. "Political Prescience: How Game Theory Solves the Paradox of Foreknowledge." *Discovering* Dune: *Essays on Frank Herbert's Epic Saga*, edited by Dominic J. Nardi and N. Trevor Brierly, McFarland, forthcoming.
Neely, Sharlotte. "The Anthropology of Dune." *The Science of Dune: An Unauthorized Exploration into the Real Science Behind Frank Herbert's Fictional Universe*, edited by Kevin R. Grazier, BenBella Books, 2008, pp. 83–88.
Nicholas, Jeffery L. "The Choices of Muad'Dib: Goods, Traditions, and Practices in the Dune Saga." *Discovering* Dune: *Essays on Frank Herbert's Epic Saga*, edited by Dominic J. Nardi and N. Trevor Brierly, McFarland, forthcoming.
Nicholas, Jeffery. "Facing the Gom Jabbar Test." *Dune and Philosophy: Weirding Way of the Mentat*, edited by Jeffery Nicholas, Open Court, 2011, pp. 3–12.
O'Reilly, Timothy. *Frank Herbert*. Frederick Ungar, 1981.
Ower, John. "Idea and Imagery in Herbert's *Dune*." *Extrapolation*, vol. 15, no. 2, 1974, pp. 129–139.
Palumbo, Donald E. "Chaos Theory, Asimov's Foundations and Robots, and Herbert's Dune: The Fractal Aesthetic of Epic Science Fiction." *Contributions to the Study of Science Fiction and Fantasy*, Number 100. Greenwood Press, 2002.
Palumbo, Donald E. *Chaos Theory, Asimov's Foundations and Robots, and Herbert's Dune: The Fractal Aesthetic of Epic Science Fiction*. Contributions to the Study of Science Fiction and Fantasy, Number 100. Greenwood Press, 2002.

Palumbo, Donald E. "The Monomyth and Chaos Theory: 'Perhaps we should believe in magic.'" *Journal of the Fantastic in the Arts*, vol. 12, no. 1, 2001, pp. 34–76.

Palumbo, Donald E. "The Monomyth as Fractal Pattern in Frank Herbert's Dune Novels." *Science Fiction Studies*, vol. 25, no. 3, 1998, pp. 433–458.

Palumbo, Donald E. "'Plots within Plots...Patterns within Patterns': Chaos-Theory Concepts and Structures in Frank Herbert's Dune Novels." *Journal of the Fantastic in the Arts*, vol. 8, no. 1, 1997, pp. 55–77.

Parkerson, Ronny W. "Semantics, General Semantics, and Ecology in Frank Herbert's *Dune*." *ETC: A Review of General Semantics*, vol. 55, no. 3, 1998, pp. 317–328.

Parkerson, Ronny W. "Semantics, General Semantics, and Ecology in Frank Herbert's *Dune*." *ETC: A Review of General Semantics*, vol. 67, no. 4, 2010, pp. 403–411 [update of 1998 version]

Parkinson, Robert C. "*Dune* – An Unfinished Tetralogy." *Extrapolation*, vol. 13, no. 1, 1971, pp. 16–24.

Pearson, Brook W.R. "Friedrich Nietzsche Goes to Space." *Dune and Philosophy: Weirding Way of the Mentat*, edited by Jeffery Nicholas, Open Court, 2011, pp. 189–205.

Pearson, Joshua. "Frank Herbert's *Dune* and the Financialization of Heroic Masculinity." *CR: The New Centennial Review*, vol. 19, no. 1, 2019, pp. 155–180.

Peden, William. "Prisoners of Prophecy: Freedom and Foreknowledge in the *Dune* Series." *Dune and Philosophy: Minds, Monads, and Muad'Dib*, edited by Kevin S. Decker, Wiley-Blackwell, forthcoming.

Phillips, Michael. "'The greatest predator ever known': The Golden Path and Political Philosophy as Ecology." *Discovering* Dune: *Essays on Frank Herbert's Epic Saga*, edited by Dominic J. Nardi and N. Trevor Brierly, McFarland, forthcoming.

Pirtle, Zachary. "Humans, Machines and an Ethics for Technology in *Dune*." *Dune and Philosophy: Minds, Monads, and Muad'Dib*, edited by Kevin S. Decker, Wiley-Blackwell, forthcoming.

Pistoi, Sergio. "My Second Sight: How Tleilaxu Eyes Changed My Life." *The Science of Dune: An Unauthorized Exploration into the Real Science Behind Frank Herbert's Fictional Universe*, edited by Kevin R. Grazier, BenBella Books, 2008, pp. 21–28.

Prieto-Pablos, Juan A. "The Ambivalent Hero of Contemporary Fantasy and Science Fiction." *Extrapolation*, vol. 32, no. 1, 1991, pp. 64–80.

Ralston, Shane. "The American Fremen." *Dune and Philosophy: Weirding Way of the Mentat*, edited by Jeffery Nicholas, Open Court, 2011, pp. 53–60.

Ray, Alice. "The Translation of *Dune*: An Encounter of Languages." *Contacts and Contrasts in Educational Contexts and Translation*, edited by Barbara Lewandowska-Tomaszczyk, Springer, 2019, pp. 183–194.

Reef, Paul. "From Sand Dunes to Planetary Ecology: Historical Perspectives on Environmental Thought and Politics in the Dune Saga." *Discovering* Dune: *Essays on Frank Herbert's Epic Saga*, edited by Dominic J. Nardi and N. Trevor Brierly, McFarland, forthcoming.

Riggs, Don. "Future and 'Progress' in *Foundation* and *Dune*." *Spectrum of the Fantastic: Selected Essays from the Sixth International Conference on the Fantastic in the Arts*, edited by Donald Palumbo, Greenwood Press, 1988, pp. 113–117.

Roberts, Adam. "Case Study: Frank Herbert, *Dune* (1965)." *Science Fiction*. Routledge, 2000, pp. 36–46.

Rogers, Brett M. "'Now Harkonnen Shall Kill Harkonnen': Aeschylus, Dynastic Violence, and Twofold Tragedies in Frank Herbert's *Dune*." *Brill's Companion to the Reception of Aeschylus*, edited by Rebecca Futo Kennedy, Brill, 2018, pp. 553–581.

Royston, Edward. "Dune and the Meta-Narrative of Power." *Discovering* Dune: *Essays on Frank Herbert's Epic Saga*, edited by Dominic J. Nardi and N. Trevor Brierly, McFarland, forthcoming.

Rudd, Amanda. "Paul's Empire: Imperialism and Assemblage Theory in Frank Herbert's *Dune*." *MOSF Journal of Science Fiction*, vol. 1, no. 1, 2016, pp. 45–57.

Ryding, Karin Christina. "The Arabic of *Dune*: Language and Landscape." *Language in Place: Stylistic Perspectives on Landscape, Place and Environment*, edited by Daniela Francesca Virdis, Elisabetta Zurru, and Ernestine Lahey, John Benjamins Publishing Company, 2021, pp. 105–123.

Schmitt-v. Muhlenfels, Astrid. "The Theme of Ecology in Frank Herbert's *Dune* Novels." *The Role of Geography in a Post-Industrial Society*, edited by Hans W. Windhorst, Vechtaer Druckerei und Verlag GmbH, 1987, pp. 27–34.

Schwartz, Susan L. "A Teaching Review of *Dune*: Religion is the Spice of Life." *Implicit Religion*, vol. 17, no. 4, 2014, pp. 533–538.

Scigaj, Leonard M. "*Prana* and the Presbyterian Fixation: Ecology and Technology in Frank Herbert's *Dune* Tetralogy." *Extrapolation*, vol. 24, no. 4, 1983, pp. 340–355.

Seger, Ges, and Kevin R. Grazier. "Suspensor of Disbelief." *The Science of Dune: An Unauthorized Exploration into the Real Science Behind Frank Herbert's Fictional Universe*, edited by Kevin R. Grazier, BenBella Books, 2008, pp. 207–216.

Semler, Stephanie. "The Golden Path of Eugenics." *Dune and Philosophy: Weirding Way of the Mentat*, edited by Jeffery Nicholas, Open Court, 2011, pp. 13–26.

Senior, William A. "Frank Herbert's Prescience: *Dune* and the Modern World." *Journal of the Fantastic in the Arts*, vol. 17, no. 4, 2007, pp. 317–320.

Siegel, Mark. "The Ecology of Politics and the Politics of Ecology in Frank Herbert's Dune." *Hugo Gernsback, Father of Modern Science Fiction, with Essays on Frank Herbert and Bram Stoker.* Borgo Press, 1988, pp. 65–75.

Simkins, Jennifer. "Resisting Tradition: The Messiah Myth and Authentic Dasein in Frank Herbert's Dune Series." *The Science Fiction Mythmakers: Religion, Science and Philosophy in Wells, Clarke, Dick and Herbert*, McFarland, 2016, pp. 121–152.

Simonetti, Nicola. "Posthuman Disability and Strategies of Containment in Frank Herbert's *Dune* Novels." *Journal of Literary & Cultural Disability Studies*, vol. 16, no. 1, 2022, pp. 77–92.

Sloan, Russell. *Evolution, The Messianic Hero, and Ecology in Frank Herbert's Dune Sequence.* 2010. University of Ulster, PhD dissertation.

Smith, John C. "Navigators and the Spacing Guild." *The Science of Dune: An Unauthorized Exploration into the Real Science Behind Frank Herbert's Fictional Universe*, edited by Kevin R. Grazier, BenBella Books, 2008a, pp. 151–166.

Smith, John C. "Stillsuit." *The Science of Dune: An Unauthorized Exploration into the Real Science Behind Frank Herbert's Fictional Universe*, edited by Kevin R. Grazier, BenBella Books, 2008b, pp. 127–142.

Smith, Tara B.M. "The Anthropocene in Frank Herbert's *Dune* Trilogy." *Foundation*, vol. 50, no. 3, 2021, pp. 62–75.

Smith, Tara B.M. "The Tangled Bank and the Ox's Tail: Reading *Dune* as a Zen Koan." 2017. University of Sydney, BA Honours Thesis.

Stratton, Susan. "The Messiah and the Greens: The Shape of Environmental Action in *Dune* and *Pacific Edge*." *Extrapolation*, vol. 42, no. 4, 2001, pp. 303–318.

Thomason, Sue. "Living Water: Archetypal Power in 'Dune' and 'The Drowned World.'" *Vector*, vol. 37, no. 119, 1984, pp. 33–34.

Touponce, William. *Frank Herbert.* Twayne Publishers, 1988.

Tranter, Kieran. "Dune, Modern Law, and the Alchemy of Death and Time." *Living in Technical Legality: Science Fiction and Law as Technology.* Edinburgh University Press, 2018, pp. 43–75.

Vereb, Zach. "Thinking like a Desert: Environmental Philosophy and *Dune*." *Dune and Philosophy: Minds, Monads, and Muad'Dib*, edited by Kevin S. Decker, Wiley-Blackwell, forthcoming.

Weyant, Curtis A. "'I suggest you may be human': Humanity and Human Action in *Dune*." *Discovering Dune: Essays on Frank Herbert's Epic Saga*, edited by Dominic J. Nardi and N. Trevor Brierly, McFarland, forthcoming.

Williams, Kevin. "Belief Is the Mind-Killer: The Bene Gesserit's Transcendental Pragmatism." *Discovering Dune: Essays on Frank Herbert's Epic Saga*, edited by Dominic J. Nardi and N. Trevor Brierly, McFarland, forthcoming.

Williams, Kevin C. "Communicative Action in Frank Herbert's Dune." *Integrative Explorations: Journal of Culture and Consciousness*, vol. 7 & 8, 2003a, pp. 151–172.

Williams, Kevin C. "Imperialism & Globalization: Lessons from Frank Herbert's Dune." *Reconstruction: Studies in Contemporary Culture*, vol. 3, no. 3, 2003b.

Williams, Kevin C. *The Wisdom of the Sand: Philosophy and Frank Herbert's Dune.* Hampton Press, 2013.

Womack, Caroline. "He Who Controls Knowledge Controls the Universe: Leto II and the Golden Path." *Discovering* Dune: *Essays on Frank Herbert's Epic Saga*, edited by Dominic J. Nardi and N. Trevor Brierly, McFarland, forthcoming.

Zaki, Hoda M. "Orientalism in Science Fiction." *Food for Our Grandmothers: Writings by Arab-American and Arab-Canadian Feminists*, edited by Joanna Kadi, South End Press, 1994, pp. 181–187.

Zeender, Marie-Noelle. "The 'Moi-peau' of Leto II in Herbert's Atreides Saga." *Science Fiction Studies*, vol. 22, no. 2, 1995, pp. 226–233.

Index

A
Ace Books, 4
Achilles, 94
Adaptations, 6
Aeschylus, 72
Al-Azhar University, 29
Alien, 6
Analog, 4
Anirul, 85
Apollo, 2, 72
Appendix, 4, 29, 38, 43, 74, 79, 90
Arabic language, 28, 30, 90, 91
Arabs, 12, 28, 29, 71
Archetypes, 7, 51, 56, 64, 65, 68, 74, 93
Army-McCarthy hearings, 7
Arrakis, *see* Dune (planet)
Artemis, 2, 72
Asimov, Isaac, 3, 5, 93
Astounding, 4
Atreides, Alia, 30, 56, 70, 72, 84, 92, 94
Atreides, Duke Leto, 2, 20, 25, 67, 72, 85, 86
Atreides, Paul, 4, 8, 10–12, 22, 23, 26–30, 38, 40, 41, 44, 50–52, 54, 55, 57–59, 64–74, 78, 80, 81, 83, 84, 86, 87, 90–95

B
Ballard, J.G., 5
Beat poets, 53
Beauvoir, Simone de, 14, 95
Bedouin, 12, 39, 91
Bene Gesserit, 7, 8, 10, 11, 14, 21, 22, 27–30, 43, 51–58, 64, 65, 68–70, 73, 75, 78, 79, 81, 82, 85, 86, 93–95
Blanch, Lesley, 29
Breeding program, 44, 58, 64, 68–70, 75, 79, 82, 85, 93, 95
Buddhism, 27, 53, 56
  Mahayana, 53
  Theravada, 53
  Vajrayana, 53
  Zen, 14, 50, 53

Butler, Samuel, 21
Butlerian Jihad, 21, 52, 70, 94

C
Caladan, 25, 38, 64, 92
Campbell, John W., 4
Campbell, Joseph, 64
Carson, Rachel, 2, 36
Catholicism, 7, 14, 15, 21, 27, 78, 79
Chani, 67, 79, 80, 84, 87
Chapterhouse: Dune, 11
Children of Dune, 11
Chilton, 4
CHOAM, *see* Combine Honnete Ober Advancer Mercantiles
Christianity, 90
Civil rights movement, 13
Cold War, 9, 12, 14
Collective unconscious, 7, 56, 93
Colonialism, 22, 23, 41
Combine Honnete Ober Advancer Mercantiles (CHOAM), 22, 23
Consciousness, 50, 52–60, 68, 70
  altered states of, 14, 53
Cordon, Guy, 7
Counterculture, 3
Crysknife, 39

D
Descartes, René, 52, 95
Desert, 2, 8, 12, 37–39, 44–46, 90–92
Dick, Philip K., 56
Dinner party, 40, 51
The Dispossessed, 45
A Door into Ocean, 5
The Dragon in the Sea, 9
Drugs, 2, 14, 15, 53, 55–58, 60, 69
Dune (planet), 2, 25, 38, 39, 43, 44, 71, 92
Dune Messiah, 4, 11
"Dune World," 4

E
East, 2, 9, 12, 14
Eastern philosophies, 52, 53, 56
Ecologist, 2, 36, 40, 43–46, 73
Ecology, 2, 6, 8–10, 36, 37, 39–46, 74, 90, 91
Ecosystem, 37, 38, 40, 42, 45
Emperor Shaddam IV, 20, 22, 25, 82, 84, 85, 87, 90
Environment, 11, 14, 37, 41, 43–46, 90, 92
Environmentalism, 2, 36, 45
Epic tradition, 2, 72, 93, 94
Epigraphs, 64, 90
Erewhon, 21

F
Fedaykin, 65, 80
The Feminine Mystique, 14
Feminism, 14, 82, 88
Fenring, Count Hasimir, 86
Fenring, Lady Margot, 54, 82
Feudal, 20, 31, 78, 79, 84
Foundation series, 5, 93
Frank Herbert's Children of Dune, 6
Frank Herbert's Dune, 6
Fremen, 22, 23, 27–30, 39–41, 43, 44, 64–66, 68, 70, 71, 73, 78, 80, 81, 83, 84, 86, 90–92, 95
Friedan, Betty, 14

G
General semantics, 8
Genetics, 11, 56, 58, 68, 69, 75, 79, 82, 85, 87
God Emperor of Dune, 11
The Godmakers, 10
Gom jabbar, 51, 54, 84
Greek mythology, 2, 72, 94
Guild, Spacing, 20, 57, 72, 94

H

Halleck, Gurney, 65
Hansen, Howard, 8
Harkonnen, Baron Vladimir, 12, 20, 22, 24, 26, 57, 67, 71, 72, 84, 86, 92, 93
Harkonnen, Feyd-Rautha, 24, 54, 65, 68, 72, 82, 92
Harkonnen, Rabban, 23, 24
Harrison, John, 6
Hawat, Thufir, 55, 82
Hayakawa, S.I., 8
Heidegger, Martin, 95
Heinlein, Robert, 3, 5, 60, 87
Herbert, Beverly (Stuart), 7, 8
Herbert, Brian, 9
Herbert, Bruce, 9
Herbert, Penny, 8
Heretics of Dune, 11
Hero, 3–5, 13, 25, 38, 40, 44, 45, 51, 58, 64, 65, 67–70, 72–75, 87, 88, 90, 92, 94
 criticism of the, 11, 26, 44
 journey of the, 10, 50, 56, 57, 64, 65, 68, 72, 87
The Hero with a Thousand Faces, 64
Hinduism, 53
Hoh, *see* Quileute Nation
House of Atreus, 2, 72
Hugo Award, 4

I

Ibn Khaldun, 22, 29
Idaho, Duncan, 65
Iliad, 72, 93
Imagery, 92
Imperialism, 22, 23, 41
Irulan, Princess, 64, 67, 82, 86, 90, 92
Islam, 27, 28, 30, 70, 71, 78, 80, 90

J

Jamis, 65, 71, 86
Jaspers, Karl, 95
Jessica, 26–30, 41, 50, 52, 54–56, 65, 68, 69, 71, 73, 78, 80–83, 85–87, 90, 92, 94, 95
Jesuits, 7, 27
Jesus, 27
Jihad, 26, 28, 31, 44, 70–72, 94
Jodorowsky, Alejandro, 6
John the Baptist, 28, 40, 73
Jordan, Robert, 5
Jung, Carl, 56, 69

K

Kennedy, John F., 12
Kwisatz Haderach, 58, 64, 69, 70, 79, 85, 87, 94
Kynes, Pardot, 40, 42, 43, 73

L

Lady Jessica, *see* Jessica
Landsraad, 20
Language, 7
Lawrence of Arabia, *see* Lawrence, T.E.
Lawrence of Arabia (film), 12
Lawrence, T.E., 12
Le Guin, Ursula K., 45, 56
Leto (of Greek mythology), 2, 72
Liet-Kynes, 28, 30, 40–44, 66, 71, 73, 95
Lisan al-Gaib, 30, 73
Litany against Fear, 55
The Lord of the Rings, 3, 4
Lucas, George, 5
Lynch, David, 6

M

Macek, Carl, 5

Machiavelli, Niccolò, 24
Machiavellianism, 24, 26
Mahdi, 27, 28, 73
Marcus, Wanna, 57
Mars trilogy, 5, 45
Martin, Henry, 8
Masculinity, 65, 66, 75, 87
McCarthy, Joseph, 7
Meditation, 53
Mentats, 57, 67, 68, 70, 85, 94, 95
Messiah, 5, 8, 10, 27–31, 38, 70–73, 75, 78, 86, 87
Middle East, 12, 14, 23, 28, 30, 38, 41, 90, 91
Milton, John, 93
Missionaria Protectiva, 27, 29, 30, 80, 87, 93, 95
Mohiam, Reverend Mother Gaius Helen, 51, 54, 55, 64, 67, 68, 70, 81, 86, 93
Monomyth, *see* Hero
Muad'Dib, 28, 30, 64, 90
Murīdīs, 71

N
Narrator, 50, 51
Native Americans, 8, 39, 91
Nebula Award, 4
Nietzsche, Friedrich, 95
Nuns, 27, 79

O
Odysseus, 94
Odyssey, 93
Oil, 2, 9, 12, 14, 15, 23, 29, 41, 90
OPEC, *see* Organization of the Petroleum Exporting Countries
Orange Catholic Bible, 27
Oresteia, 72

Organization of the Petroleum Exporting Countries (OPEC), 12, 23
Orientalism, 29
Ottoman Sultan-Caliph Mehmed v Reshad, 71

P
Paradise Lost, 93
Parkinson, Flora, 8
Planetologist, Imperial, *see* Liet-Kynes
Postcolonialism, 91
Posthumanism, 94
Prana-bindu, 53, 54, 56, 68
Prescience, 10, 11, 57, 64, 69, 70, 73, 87, 93, 94
"The Priests of Psi," 10
The Prince, 24, 25
"The Prophet of Dune," 4
Psychology, 60, 92
  Freudian, 7, 92
  Jungian, 7, 9, 10, 92, 93

Q
Quileute Nation, 8, 91
Qur'anic verse, 29

R
Ramallo, Reverend Mother, 55, 69
Religion, 2, 11, 27–29, 31, 71, 73, 78–80, 91, 93
Reproduction, 81, 82, 85, 87
Robinson, Kim Stanley, 5, 45
Robotech series, 5

S
The Sabres of Paradise, 29
Sand dunes, 8, 36, 38, 41, 92

Sandworms, 2, 26, 28, 30, 38, 39, 43, 45, 46, 58, 90, 92, 93
Sanskrit, 54, 56
Sardaukar, 22, 39, 68, 84
Sayyadina, 80
Science fiction
　Golden Age, 3–5
　hard, 5
　New Wave, 5, 60
　soft, 5, 60, 75
Scott, Ridley, 6
The Second Sex, 14
Second Vatican Council, 14
Seven Pillars of Wisdom, 12
Shadout Mapes, 28, 80
Shakespeare, 1, 24
Silent Spring, 2, 36, 37
Slattery, Ralph and Irene, 7
Slonczewski, Joan, 5
Spice, 12, 21–25, 38, 39, 41, 44–46, 53, 55, 57, 58, 69, 70, 90, 92, 94
Star Wars, 5
Stilgar, 8, 66, 73, 80, 81, 83, 84, 86
Stillsuits, 39
Stranger in a Strange Land, 3, 5, 60, 87
Suk Medical School, 57
Suzuki, D.T., 53
Symbols, 92

T
Taoism, 27, 56
Terraforming, 2, 41, 42, 44, 45
Tiresias, 94
Tolkien, J.R.R., 3, 4, 31, 45
Translations, 91
Truthsayer, 21, 86

21st Century Sub, see *The Dragon in the Sea*

U
Unconscious, 10, 54, 56, 58, 69, 93
Under Pressure, see *The Dragon in the Sea*
Usul, 30

V
Van Vogt, A.E., 75
Vedanta, 53
Villeneuve, Denis, 6
Voice, 55, 68, 75, 81, 82, 93
Vries, Piter de, 24

W
Water, 2, 7, 38–41, 43, 45, 80, 83, 86, 92
Water of Life, 55, 70, 80, 86, 92
Watts, Alan, 53
Weirding way, 65, 83, 86
West, 2, 9, 12, 14
Western philosophies, 52, 53
The Wheel of Time series, 5
Whole Earth Catalog, 3
World-building, 4, 6, 45, 90, 91
The Word for World Is Forest, 45

Y
Yaitanes, Greg, 6
Yoga, 14, 53
Yueh, Dr. Wellington, 26, 57

GPSR Compliance
The European Union's (EU) General Product Safety Regulation (GPSR) is a set of rules that requires consumer products to be safe and our obligations to ensure this.

If you have any concerns about our products, you can contact us on

ProductSafety@springernature.com

In case Publisher is established outside the EU, the EU authorized representative is:

Springer Nature Customer Service Center GmbH
Europaplatz 3
69115 Heidelberg, Germany

www.ingramcontent.com/pod-product-compliance
Ingram Content Group UK Ltd.
Pitfield, Milton Keynes, MK11 3LW, UK
UKHW021251180426
11946UKWH00004B/74